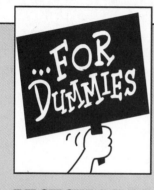

TM

BESTSELLING BOOK SERIES

References for the Rest of Us!®

Are you intimidated and confused by computers? Do you find that traditional manuals are overloaded with technical details you'll never use? Do your friends and family always call you to fix simple problems on their PCs? Then the For Dummies® computer book series from Wiley Publishing, Inc. is for you.

For Dummies books are written for those frustrated computer users who know they aren't really dumb but find that PC hardware, software, and indeed the unique vocabulary of computing make them feel helpless. For Dummies books use a lighthearted approach, a down-to-earth style, and even cartoons and humorous icons to dispel computer novices' fears and build their confidence. Lighthearted but not lightweight, these books are a perfect survival guide for anyone forced to use a computer.

Already, millions of satisfied readers agree. They have made For Dummies books the #1 introductory level computer book series and have written asking for more. So, if you're looking for the most fun and easy way to learn about computers, look to For Dummies books to give you a helping hand.

Wiley Publishing, Inc.

5/09

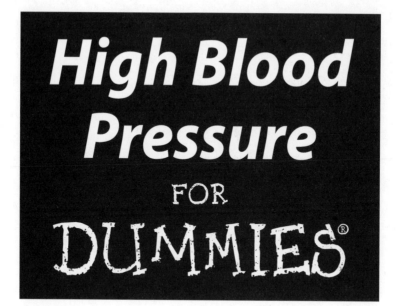

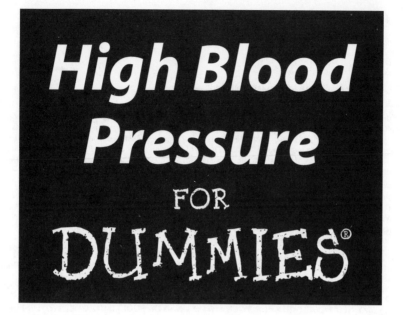

High Blood Pressure

FOR

DUMMIES®

by Alan L. Rubin, MD

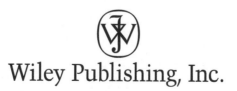

Wiley Publishing, Inc.

Best-Selling Books • Digital Downloads • e-Books • Answer Networks • e-Newsletters • Branded Web Sites • e-Learning

High Blood Pressure For Dummies®

Published by
Wiley Publishing, Inc.
909 Third Avenue
New York, NY 10022
www.wiley.com

Copyright ® 2002 by Wiley Publishing, Inc., Indianapolis, Indiana

Published simultaneously in Canada

For general information on our other products and services or to obtain technical support, please contact our Customer Care Department within the U.S. at 800-762-2974, outside the U.S. at 317-572-3993, or fax 317-572-4002.

Wiley also publishes its books in a variety of electronic formats. Some content that appears in print may not be available in electronic books.

Library of Congress Control Number: 2002106049

ISBN: 0-7645-5424-7

Printed in the United States of America

10 9 8 7 6 5 4

1B/RS/QX/QS/IN

About the Author

Alan L. Rubin, MD has been managing and studying high blood pressure for three decades. He is a best-selling author whose previous books, *Diabetes For Dummies, Diabetes Cookbook For Dummies,* and *Thyroid For Dummies* have been major successes. Letters of praise from numerous readers verify the important role that his books have played in their lives. His books provide the latest information on every aspect of their subject while being written in an easy-to-understand format that's full of humor and wisdom.

Dr. Rubin has practiced endocrinology in San Francisco since 1973. He teaches doctors, medical students, and nonprofessionals through classes, lectures, and articles. He has been on numerous radio and television shows, answering questions about diabetes, thyroid disease, and high blood pressure. He serves as a consultant to many pharmaceutical companies and companies that make products for high blood pressure.

Dedication

This book is dedicated to my mother Edith. Besides the fact that I would not exist were it not for her (with a little help from my father Julius), she always let me know in no uncertain terms that I could do anything I set my mind to. This is the fourth *For Dummies* book I have written, and that knowledge helped to get me through each one. Not only did she give me total verbal approval, but she backed it up by making sure I got a great undergraduate education at Brandeis University and medical education at New York University School of Medicine. Most important of all, she made sure I knew that I was loved.

Acknowledgments

Unlike a baby, this book has more than two parents. The people who worked on it are dedicated, bright, and cheerful and they deserve a standing ovation. The original concept belongs to Kathy Nebenhaus who was Lifestyles Publisher when the book began and is now Vice President of Professional and Trade Publishing at Wiley Books. Acquisitions Editor Natasha Graf was tremendously helpful throughout the writing of the book, smoothing all the rough edges that inevitably surround such a major project. Project Editor Alissa Schwipps had a very clear idea of how the book would best serve its readers and offered many helpful suggestions to accomplish this. Copyeditor Esmeralda St. Clair made sure that my words, my sentences, and my paragraphs followed the rules of the English language. Last but definitely not least, Dr. Dorothee Perloff was the technical editor for this book, utilizing her great knowledge of this subject to assure that my information is consistent with current medical practice. To all of them, I owe major thanks.

Publisher's Acknowledgments

We're proud of this book; please send us your comments through our Dummies Online Registration Form located at www.dummies.com.

Some of the people who helped bring this book to market include the following:

Acquisitions, Editorial, and Media Development

Project Editor: Alissa Schwipps

Acquisitions Editor: Natasha Graf

Copy Editor: Esmeralda St. Clair

Technical Editor: Dorothee Perloff, MD

Editorial Manager: Jennifer Ehrlich

Editorial Assistant: Nívea C. Strickland

Cover Photo: Alan L. Rubin, MD

Production

Project Coordinator: Dale White

Layout and Graphics: Scott Bristol, Clint Lahnene, LeAndra Johnson, Brent Savage, Jacque Schneider, Betty Schulte

Special Art: Kathryn Born, Medical Illustrator

Proofreaders: Andy Hollandbeck, Susan Moritz, Angel Perez, Carl Pierce, TECHBOOKS Production Services

Indexer: TECHBOOKS Production Services

Publishing and Editorial for Consumer Dummies

  Diane Graves Steele, Vice President and Publisher, Consumer Dummies

  Joyce Pepple, Acquisitions Director, Consumer Dummies

  Kristin A. Cocks, Product Development Director, Consumer Dummies

  Michael Spring, Vice President and Publisher, Travel

  Brice Gosnell, Publishing Director, Travel

  Suzanne Jannetta, Editorial Director, Travel

Publishing for Technology Dummies

  Andy Cummings, Acquisitions Director

Composition Services

  Gerry Fahey, Executive Director of Production Services

  Debbie Stailey, Director of Composition Services

Contents at a Glance

Cartoons at a Glance

By Rich Tennant

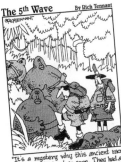

"It's a mystery why this ancient race of people died out so soon. They had an abundance of food available. The jungle here is filled with cookie bushes and the streams are full of bacon fish."

page 7

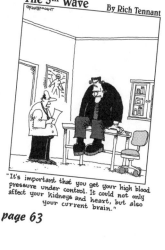

"It's important that you get your high blood pressure under control. It could not only affect your kidneys and heart, but also your current brain."

page 63

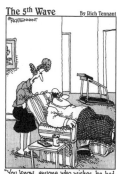

"You know, anyone who wishes he had a remote control for his exercise equipment is missing the idea of exercise equipment."

page 115

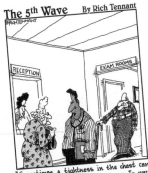

"Sometimes a tightness in the chest can be a sign of high blood pressure. In your husband's case, however, I just loosened his belt a little."

page 225

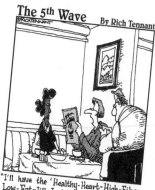

"I'll have the 'Healthy-Heart-High-Fiber-Low-Fat-I'll-Just-Have-A-Bite-Of-My-Neighbor's-Eggs-Benedict Breakfast'."

page 263

Cartoon Information:
Fax: 978-546-7747
E-Mail: richtennant@the5thwave.com
World Wide Web: www.the5thwave.com

Table of Contents

Part IV: Investigating Special Populations 225

Chapter 14: The Elderly 227

Introduction

When I was growing up, my mother often used the pressure cooker to make dinner in a hurry. The idea was that if you cooked food at higher pressures, the food would get done faster. High blood pressure in people is like that. If you permit yourself to have high blood pressure, you'll get done faster. What do I mean by *done?* I am talking about all the medical complications, such as heart attack, stroke, and kidney failure, as well as the shortened life span of people with poorly treated or untreated high blood pressure.

High blood pressure, or *hypertension,* as doctors like to call it, affects more than 50 million adults in the United States and between 15 and 25 percent of the rest of the world according to the World Health Organization. That means that if you're in a room with three other adults, one of the four of you probably has high blood pressure. One major problem is that a third of the time that person is unaware that she has the condition. High blood pressure is generally free of symptoms until it has time to do its damage over ten or more years. That's why it's often known as the "silent killer."

A second major problem is that of the other two-thirds who have high blood pressure and know it: 15 percent are untreated, 26 percent are on inadequate treatment for it, and only 27 percent are receiving adequate treatment.

Translating percentages into numbers, around 37.5 million Americans are at risk from the complications of high blood pressure because they're unaware of the presence of the disease, not being treated, or being treated inadequately. The situation in most other countries is even worse.

For decades, the crusade to bring this vast problem under control seemed to be making great progress. In the last few years, however, this trend is reversing. A major investment of time, energy, and money is needed to lower high blood pressure.

Like diabetes, high blood pressure is a lifestyle disease. It tends to occur in more affluent nations where food is plentiful and hard manual labor is done less often. This is both a problem and a challenge. On the one hand, affluent societies don't want to give up their benefits. On the other, the more fortunate want to enjoy their blessings without destroying themselves.

In this book, you can find everything that you need to know to understand high blood pressure — its causes, its consequences, and its treatment. You'll soon come to realize that high blood pressure is easily recognized and just as easily treated. Sure, great drugs are available for treating high blood pressure, but no lowering of blood pressure with drugs comes without cost in the form of drug side effects, as well as the expense of doctor visits and medications. Far more benign and less costly is a dedication on your part to change the lifestyle habits that lead to high blood pressure. You can find all the necessary information on how to do that as you read the chapters of this book, especially Part III.

I always like to have a bottom line in my books, and this one is no exception. The bottom line is that you never have to suffer any of the consequences of high blood pressure. You have it within your brain and your body to prevent it or successfully treat high blood pressure should you discover that you have it. Imagine if all the people with high blood pressure heeded this advice and got theirs under control. About 250,000 lives a year would be saved, not to mention a much larger number who suffer but don't die. And that's in the United States alone, not to mention the rest of the world.

If you read any of my previous books, *Diabetes For Dummies, Diabetes Cookbook For Dummies,* or *Thyroid For Dummies,* you know that I use humor to get my point across, a technique that characterizes the *For Dummies* series. I want to emphasize that I'm not trying to trivialize anyone's suffering by being comic about it. The work of Norman Cousins (who wrote a book called *Anatomy of an Illness as Perceived by the Patient* [Bantam Doubleday Dell] that showed how he cured himself of an "incurable" disease using humor) and others has shown that humor has healing properties. A positive attitude is far more conducive to a positive outcome than is a negative attitude.

About This Book

No one expects that you'll read this book from cover to cover. Because the first few chapters are a general introduction to high blood pressure, you may start in Part I, but if you prefer to go right to the treatment or the special concerns of different populations, by all means, do so.

It's important that each chapter stand alone. You don't have to skip back to Chapter 3 to understand Chapter 12. You don't have to start at the beginning to understand the end. It's not a novel, after all, but a tool to help you manage your high blood pressure. (Though some people may think of high blood pressure as a villain.)

Conventions Used in This Book

As much as I would love to use all nonscientific terms in this book, if I do so, you and your doctor will be speaking two different languages. Therefore, I use the scientific term, but I explain it with simple language the first time you see it.

As for using the term *high blood pressure* or the word *hypertension,* in this case and in all cases, I use the simpler term — high blood pressure. This seems to be the trend, and I think it's a good trend so long as the information that the word provides is accurate and comprehensive.

What You Don't Have to Read

Throughout the book, shaded areas (called sidebars) contain material that's interesting but not essential to your understanding. If you don't care to go so deeply into a subject, skip the sidebars. You'll understand everything else.

Assumptions

This book makes no assumptions about what you know. All new terms are explained. If you already know a great deal, you'll find new information that adds to your knowledge. Key points are always marked clearly for you. You probably fall into one of the following categories:

- ✔ You've been diagnosed with high blood pressure but haven't started treatment.
- ✔ You're being treated for high blood pressure but aren't happy with the results.
- ✔ You have a close friend or family member with high blood pressure.

How This Book is Organized

The book is divided into six parts to help you find out all that you want to know about high blood pressure.

Part 1: Understanding High Blood Pressure

This part is really the introduction to the subject. You'll discover the definition of high blood pressure, how to measure it correctly and how to separate essential high blood pressure, the cause of which is basically unknown, from secondary high blood pressure, which results from another disease.

Part II: Considering the Medical Consequences

High blood pressure can damage many parts of the body, but it's especially dangerous to your heart, your kidneys, and your brain. In this part, you find out exactly how the damage is done and what the results of that damage will be in these important organs.

Part III: Treating High Blood Pressure

In this part, you discover everything that's known about lowering high blood pressure after it develops. This is a highly treatable condition. First, you need to know that you have it and then what to do about it. High blood pressure treatment has definite goals. You must meet those goals, not just take a pill and assume you're "home free."

Part IV: Investigating Special Populations

Three groups of people deserve special consideration because high blood pressure acts differently and has different consequences in pregnant women, children, and the elderly. This part addresses their problems.

Part V: The Part of Tens

Like many other major medical conditions, misinformation about high blood pressure is rampant. In the part of tens, I clear up some (not all, because it accumulates faster than I can address it) of it and show you how you can take simple measures to control your blood pressure.

The pace of discovery is rapid. After this book is published, it's fixed in terms of its information until a revision is done. You need to know where to find new, accurate, and useful information about high blood pressure until I come out with my latest revision. You can find ten such places in another chapter in this part.

Just to whet your appetite and convince you that the field is not static, I also provide ten new up-to-the-minute discoveries.

Icons Used in This Book

Books in the *For Dummies* series feature icons, which direct you toward information that may be of particular interest or importance. Here's an explanation of what each icon in this book signifies:

I define medical terms where you see this icon.

When you see this icon, it means the information is essential. You want to be sure you understand it.

When you find this alongside some information, it's time to dial the doctor for help.

This icon points out important information that can save you time and energy.

This icon warns against potential problems (for example if you mix the wrong drugs).

Where to Go From Here

Where you go from here depends on your needs. If you want to understand how high blood pressure develops, head to Part I. If you or someone you know has a complication due to high blood pressure, skip to Part II. For help in treating high blood pressure using every available tool, turn to Part III. If you are pregnant or have a child or parent with high blood pressure, Part IV is your next stop. For a bird's eye view of treatment, high blood pressure mythology, and the latest discoveries, you can find that in Part V.

If you experienced something funny in connection with your high blood pressure condition, by all means, let me know about it by e-mailing me at hypertension@drrubin.com. I'll share it with the world in a future edition of this book if it's appropriate.

In any case, as my mother used to say when she gave me a present, use this book in good health.

Part I
Understanding High Blood Pressure

The 5th Wave   By Rich Tennant

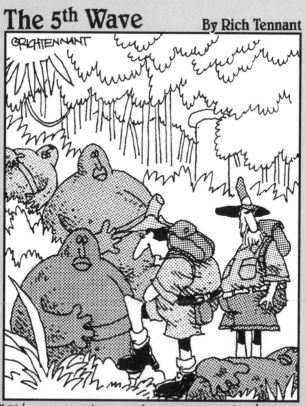

"It's a mystery why this ancient race of people died out so soon. They had an abundance of food available. The jungle here is filled with cookie bushes and the streams are full of bacon fish."

In this part . . .

What are those two numbers your doctor gives you after measuring your blood pressure? In this part, I answer that question and describe the correct technique for taking blood pressure at home or in your doctor's office. I also discuss who is most at risk for developing high blood pressure and what you need to know about secondary high blood pressure.

Chapter 1

Getting Acquainted with High Blood Pressure

*I*f you have high blood pressure, you're in good (if not terribly healthy) company. Fifty million Americans (one in four adults) have high blood pressure. A list of the people in this country with high blood pressure would read like a Who's Who. The problem is that, without proper treatment, many of those people will be on a list of Who Was Who sooner than they may want. Don't let yourself or a loved one get on the Who Was Who list without a fight.

You can do so much about high blood pressure. First, you can prevent it. If your blood pressure is already high, you can control it. But before you can do these things, you need to know what high blood pressure is and how you measure it. Then understanding what's known about how high blood pressure occurs and how it's treated is important. This book is your blood pressure companion. It provides you with a solid understanding of your blood pressure: how it affects your body — organ by organ, who is at risk, how you can prevent it, and how you can treat high blood pressure after it's properly diagnosed. I also discuss the effects of high blood pressure in children, pregnant women, and the elderly. Lastly, you'll find out about myths associated with high blood pressure and the latest related discoveries in the Part of Tens of this book.

As you'll discover, a few simple alterations to your lifestyle can prevent high blood pressure. My hope is that as you read the information in this book, you'll be spurred on to make these changes, not just now but continuing into the future. High blood pressure is a chronic disease. You may lower your blood pressure in the short term, but the goal is long-term control to prevent other medical consequences (discussed in Part II).

Take charge of your blood pressure now, and you won't have the fate of a health food store owner who posted a sign that read, "Closed due to illness."

Understanding Your Cardiovascular System

To understand how elevated blood pressure affects your overall health, it's important to understand what makes Thumper tick — well, pump. Your cardiovascular system — your heart, arteries, veins capillaries, and the blood that fills them — nourishes your body and connects each part of the body to every other part. The cardiovascular system carries

- ✓ **Food** in the form of carbohydrates, protein, fat, vitamins, and minerals and brought in through the gastrointestinal tract to every organ in the body.

- ✓ **Oxygen,** brought in through the lungs and dissolved in the blood, to organs far from the lungs.

- ✓ **Waste,** a normal product of your body's metabolism that results from the many chemical reactions that are taking place in your body. For example, the cardiovascular system carries carbon dioxide to the lungs and the other waste products to the liver and kidneys.

Pressure must exist to push the blood through the cardiovascular system. Otherwise, on standing, your blood would pool in your legs and stay there due to gravity. Just as your modern household water supply gets to you because pressure is pushing water through the pipes, the blood gets to your brain because pressure is allowing it to defy gravity and rise from the heart. The heart muscle, the source of this pressure, squeezes out the blood forcefully so the blood not only defies gravity but goes through the smallest passageways (the capillaries) that allow for exchanges, such as the release of oxygen and the uptake of carbon dioxide between the blood and the tissues through which it's passing.

When essential body organs, such as the kidneys, don't receive enough pressure to allow them to function properly, they signal the heart to pump harder. But what's good for the kidneys may not be good for the brain or the blood vessels themselves. That's when the consequences of high blood pressure occur (described in Part II).

Taking Your Pressure and Understanding the Measurement

When the nurse in your doctor's office measures your blood pressure, she puts a funny-looking contraption with a cuff, a gauge, and some Velcro around your arm. She pumps the cuff up with air, listens with the stethoscope, turns a screw to release the air pressure, and then writes down a couple numbers in your chart. Then your doctor re-enters and says that those numbers are "good" or "not so good." What's that contraption? What's the meaning of those numbers? Why does it seem to have such a profound effect on your life? Good questions. That "contraption" is a *sphygmomanometer.* And, for example, when your doctor says that your blood pressure is "135 over 85," the first number (135) is the *systolic blood pressure;* the second number (85) is the *diastolic blood pressure.* In Chapter 2, I discuss what each pressure measures and what each number means, as well as why this has a serious effect on your life.

Examining the Risk Factors for High Blood Pressure

A tremendous effort has been made to understand the cause of high blood pressure and what populations are at risk of developing the disease. Numerous unalterable factors affect blood pressure (such as age, sex, ethnic background, and family history), and to some extent, how these factors can contribute to high blood pressure is understood. But which of these factors is the major factor is unknown. I discuss these risk factors in detail in Chapter 3.

Certain changeable factors (such as diet, exercise routine, and stress) can also place you at risk of developing high blood pressure. Ask yourself the following questions:

- Am I less active than I could be in my day-to-day routine?
- Am I overweight?
- Do I eat many salty foods?
- Do I have a stressful lifestyle?
- Do I smoke? Drink?

If you answered "Yes" to any one of these questions, then you're at risk of developing high blood pressure. The more questions that you answer in the affirmative, the greater your odds are for developing high blood pressure. If you decrease the stress in your life and keep a rein on these changeable factors, you can decrease the possibility of developing high blood pressure. I discuss high blood pressure prevention further in Chapter 3.

Ninety-five percent of high blood pressure is categorized as *essential high blood pressure* (but "primary high blood pressure" would be a better term) because what's causing the elevated pressure is unknown. In all other cases, a specific disease is identifiable that, when treated, usually normalizes the blood pressure. This is *secondary high blood pressure*. I discuss some causes of secondary high blood pressure (such as kidney disease and adrenal gland tumors) in Chapter 4. I also discuss special at-risk populations, including the elderly, children, and pregnant women, in Part IV.

Reviewing the Consequences of High Blood Pressure

High blood pressure can wreak havoc on your heart, kidneys, and brain, if untreated. Heart attacks and/or heart failure may be the major consequence for your heart (see Chapter 5). Kidney failure may affect your kidneys (see Chapter 6). A brain attack (stroke) may destroy important brain tissue and the movements it controls in the body (see Chapter 7).

Deaths due to these conditions do occur, but the greater majority of those who have serious conditions resulting from high blood pressure suffer debilitating illness. Of those who survive a massive heart attack, kidney failure, or brain attack, many require the care of others for the rest of their lives.

Most of this sickness and death due to high blood pressure is preventable. Part III gives you all the tools you need to accomplish this. It may be costly in terms of your time and your resources, but the savings in freedom from illness and a longer life is worth it

Treating High Blood Pressure

Treating high blood pressure involves making use of all the tools discussed in Part III. Switching from a diet that promotes high blood pressure to a diet that lowers blood pressure — from a diet that's high in salt and fats to a diet that emphasizes grains, fruits, and vegetables, changes your lifestyle for the better.

Then add regular exercise to this. A program of daily aerobic exercise (see Chapter 12) is not excessive, but it should be done at least four times a week.

Next, eliminate the poisons, such as tobacco, excessive alcohol, and some caffeine (see Chapter 11). At this point, you may have done enough to lower your pressure to normal. If not, you have the option of adding one or more drugs (see Chapter 13). Drugs shouldn't be a substitute for improvements in your lifestyle, but *in addition* to lifestyle changes.

Cardiac output and peripheral resistance

An increase in blood volume creates an increase in cardiac output. An increase in blood volume results from salt intake, for example, which causes water retention. More blood volume may be present in the central part of the body and less in the peripheral part. The body doesn't permit the cardiac output to remain elevated. It lowers the cardiac output by increasing the peripheral resistance. The blood vessels constrict so that too much blood doesn't flow through the tissues. This rise in peripheral resistance leads to increased blood pressure.

A minor alteration in body chemistry may be enough to cause persistent high blood pressure. For example, a slight increase in angiotensin II, a hormone produced when the kidney detects a low blood pressure, may cause thickening and narrowing of the blood vessels that then leads to sustained high blood pressure. Other hormones, called *growth factors,* can lead to narrow arteries and increased peripheral resistance as well.

On the other hand, a chemical called *nitric oxide,* made in the endothelial cells that line the inside of the blood vessels, is the most potent cause of widening in blood vessels. If anything blocks the production of nitric oxide, the blood pressure rises. It's known that nitric oxide is reduced in essential high blood pressure, and this may be a further cause of the increased peripheral resistance.

Focusing on Children, Pregnant Women, and the Elderly

Special features must be considered when evaluating and treating high blood pressure in children, pregnant women, and the elderly.

The elderly (discussed in Chapter 14) usually have other complicating diseases and are taking many other medications. The elderly may have special dietary requirements and respond differently to the medications they're given, if they take them at all. The elderly deserve their own chapter.

Likewise, children have peculiarities that must be addressed (see Chapter 15). Growing, maturing, and subject to all the problems of relating to their peers, kids certainly don't want to be sick or thought of as "sick." Diagnosis and treatment of high blood pressure in children is challenging to say the least. Those of you who are parents understand how difficult life can be for you and your child whenever there is any deviation from "normal." A separate chapter focuses on the problems of children with high blood pressure.

Throughout pregnancy, the pregnant woman is making new hormones while her body is undergoing major changes. The high blood pressure that occasionally develops as a direct complication of pregnancy can harm both a mother and her unborn baby. Her special needs are addressed in Chapter 16, where you can also find information on how menopause affects blood pressure.

Staying Informed

The Part of Tens chapters in this book give you helpful tips on reducing your blood pressure, debunking blood pressure myths, and finding the latest information on high blood pressure.

In Chapter 17, you can find ten simple ways to reduce blood pressure. Individually, they each help to lower the pressure by a few millimeters of mercury. Taken together, they help you avoid the medical complications of high blood pressure and can be added to your lifestyle one step at a time or several at once if you feel up to it. The key is to make the changes and not fall back into old habits.

Myths about high blood pressure and its treatment are numerous. I take up only ten in Chapter 18, but I tried to find the myths that are most often believed and are most detrimental to your health. If you know of a myth that you think is damaging to many people with high blood pressure, by all means e-mail me at highbloodpressure@drrubin.com and let me know.

As in all fields of medicine that affect large numbers of people, the research on high blood pressure is enormous and ongoing. Chapter 19 introduces you to some of the latest information that could save your life. Don't miss it.

Finally, the book has a publication deadline date. Discoveries made after that date can't be in this edition (but will be in a future edition). To keep up with future developments, Chapter 20 provides the best places to look for new information. Some of it can be found on my Web site (www.drrubin.com). Or you can go there and click on the useful Web addresses in the section under high blood pressure.

All this material comes to you at a bargain price. As the sign on the farmer's gate reads: "The farmer allows walkers to cross the field for free but the bull charges."

Chapter 2

Detecting High Blood Pressure

· ·

In This Chapter

▶ Getting an accurate reading and how to do it

▶ Understanding the numbers

▶ Assessing blood pressure at home: Ambulatory readings

▶ Finding the cause and getting a thorough evaluation

· ·

Measuring blood pressure is key to diagnosing high blood pressure. You or another trained individual can take that measurement. Because everything that comes after that depends on an accurate measurement, this chapter shows you how that measurement should be done. Should you notice that your healthcare provider is not measuring your blood pressure accurately, don't hesitate to tell him. It's your life, your health, and your future that I'm talking about.

Much goes into an accurate blood pressure measurement. It requires a properly working instrument, a patient who is physically and mentally prepared for the measurement, and someone who knows how to measure blood pressure properly. And after it's done properly, it needs to be done again to be sure of the measurement.

After a diagnosis of high blood pressure is made, the way that the evaluation proceeds determines whether the doctor discovers a secondary cause for the high blood pressure (see Chapter 4). The proper evaluation is provided at the end of this chapter so that you can confirm that no stone is left unturned.

Focusing on the Fundamentals

The instrument that measures your blood pressure is a *sphygmomanometer* (pronounced sfig-mo-ma-*nom*-et-er, so why don't they spell it that way?). However, I think "blood pressure gauge" is clearer and easier to pronounce. I hope that you don't mind if I call it that from here on in.

Mercury versus aneroid gauges

The mercury blood pressure gauge is still considered the "gold standard" for blood pressure measurement. Very little can cause this device to malfunction. The column of mercury is all that moves on this type of gauge. The mercury blood pressure gauge is becoming less common, however, because mercury is toxic and has the potential to contaminate the environment.

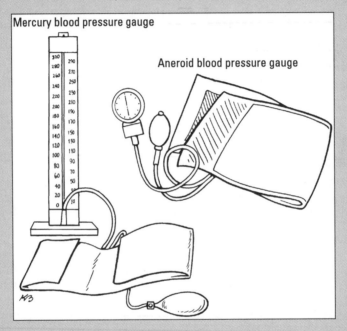

Mercury blood pressure gauge

Aneroid blood pressure gauge

An alternative blood pressure gauge that's rising in popularity is the aneroid blood pressure gauge — a spring-gauge model that uses air pressure to move a needle above a scale. Each degree the needle moves represents one millimeter of mercury. This type of gauge is inexpensive and easier to transport than the mercury blood pressure gauge.

Both models require a certain degree of upkeep. When using the mercury blood pressure gauge, check periodically to be sure that the top of the column is at zero before pressure is added and that the mercury moves freely.

When using the aneroid blood pressure gauge, calibrate and validate it on a regular basis at your doctor's office (at least every six months) by attaching it to the pressure system of a mercury manometer. Both gauges should read the same pressure when air is introduced. Unlike the mercury gauge, the aneroid gauge has many parts that can wear down after a period of time. But according to a Mayo Clinic study in the *Archives of Internal Medicine* (March 2001), "well-maintained aneroid devices are an accurate and useful alternative [to mercury devices]."

The blood pressure gauge consists of a cuff that goes around your arm above the elbow. The *bladder* is the part of the cuff that fills with air. A tube connects the cuff to a column of mercury (that looks like an outdoor thermometer) at one end and a rubber bulb at the other. When the rubber bulb is squeezed, the air pressure in this closed system also forces the column of mercury to rise while filling the bladder with air. Numbers along the column of mercury indicate how much pressure is present.

Taking Your Blood Pressure Correctly

Your blood pressure can be taken with a mercury blood pressure gauge, an aneroid manometer, or an electronic device for measuring the blood pressure, so long as the device has been recently calibrated and validated. (For more on the differences between mercury and aneroid blood pressure gauges, see the "Mercury versus aneroid gauges" sidebar in this chapter. I discuss electronic gauges in the "Taking Your Blood Pressure at Home" section later in this chapter.) With rare exceptions, blood pressure gauges found in supermarkets or pharmacies aren't properly maintained and shouldn't be used.

Following a few simple rules is important to get an accurate reading:

- ✔ First, don't smoke or drink alcohol or coffee within 15 minutes of a blood pressure measurement.

- ✔ Second, the length of the bladder should be 80 percent of the circumference of the upper arm. This means that heavy or very muscular people with thick arms need a larger bladder, while children need a smaller bladder.

- ✔ Third, your posture is important. Sit with your back supported and your elbow at about the level of your heart with your arm supported. Your legs should not be dangling. It's better if you rest for several minutes in that position before the measurement. Don't talk during the measurement.

Now to take the reading, see the following numbered steps:

1. **Leaving the cuff's lower edge about an inch above the bend of the elbow, place the cuff over your bare arm, close the cuff around the arm, and then stick the Velcro together at the ends of the cuff.**

2. **Place the earpieces of the stethoscope in your ears and place the stethoscope bell at the side of the cuff away from your heart and over the brachial artery, which is found in the inner area of your bent elbow (see Figure 2-1).**

   The *stethoscope,* a convenient device to listen for sounds at various body sites, has a point of contact known as the stethoscope's *bell.* The two earpieces at the other end of the stethoscope enable the individual taking the measurement to hear the steady "thump" in the brachial artery.

3. **Tighten the screw at the side of the rubber bulb and squeeze the bulb.**

   Air is pumped into the bulb, and thus the cuff expands.

4. **The cuff is inflated until the blood flow through your brachial artery stops.**

   With sufficient compression, the cuff cuts off blood flow through the artery, and no sound is heard in the stethoscope. The pressure in the cuff is increased rapidly to 30 millimeters of mercury above the point that no blood flow is taking place through the cuff when no sound can be heard in the stethoscope or when a pulse can no longer be felt in the wrist.

5. **Turn the screw again to loosen the valve in the bulb and to lessen the air pressure.**

   Pressure is then decreased so that the rate of drop is 2 millimeters per second. When the pressure falls to the point that blood begins to flow through the artery again, the number that the column of mercury has risen to at the first sound heard in the stethoscope is the *systolic blood pressure* (SBP), the first number in the blood pressure reading. (See the "Comprehending the Numbers" section later in this chapter.)

6. **Look at the column of mercury to see the number at that pressure point.**

7. **When the cuff decompresses to the point that blood flows freely in the artery, the sound is no longer heard in the stethoscope.**

   The number next to the top of the column of mercury when the sound ceases is the *diastolic blood pressure* (DBP), the second number in the blood pressure reading. (See the "Comprehending the Numbers" section later in this chapter.)

8. **Again, look at the column of mercury to see the number at that pressure point.**

9. **Record the SBP and the DBP numbers immediately (don't depend on memory), and note the arm (right or left) used for taking the measurement is noted.**

10. **If the first measurement is elevated, take another measurement in the same arm after 60 seconds. Then the other arm is measured.**

    The arm that has the higher blood pressure is the one that's used in the future. (They're often the same.) The average of the two measurements in the arm that supplies the more abnormal reading is considered to be the correct blood pressure.

Measure the blood pressure while the patient is in a standing position especially in the event that the patient experiences lightheadedness on standing. If a fall of 20 or more millimeters of mercury occurs in systolic blood pressure or 10 or more in diastolic blood pressure, the patient is considered to have *orthostatic hypotension,* an abnormally great fall in blood pressure with standing.

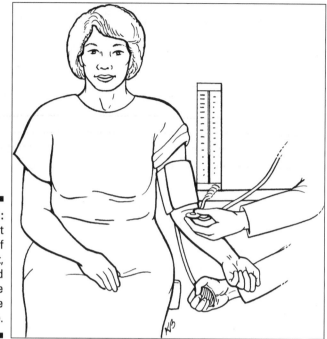

Figure 2-1:
The correct
position of
the patient,
the blood
pressure
cuff, and the
stethoscope.

If your blood pressure isn't normal, don't start any treatment on the basis of one office visit. This is treatment for life and should be done only after confirmation at a second and even a third office visit. It may even be, as shown in the next section, that your blood pressure in your doctor's office is not an accurate assessment of your blood pressure despite using entirely correct techniques. A blood pressure reading that's greater than 180/120 millimeters of mercury (mm Hg) requires immediate treatment.

Avoiding an Inaccurate Reading

When measuring blood pressure, many problems can arise that can lead to an inaccurate blood pressure reading. Because your reading may mean the difference between a lifetime of taking pills and freedom from such a task, avoiding these problems is important. Problems that interfere with an accurate reading can arise at every stage of taking a blood pressure measurement and can be due to equipment failures, faulty observation, or patient difficulties. Consider the points that follow in the next two sections when someone else takes your blood pressure or you take it yourself.

Steering clear of equipment problems

A faulty stethoscope can lead to an inaccurate blood pressure reading. To get a good reading, make sure that

✔ The earpieces aren't plugged, and sound can be heard clearly. If the earpieces are broken, replace them.

✔ The bell of the stethoscope (the part that's placed on the arm) is not cracked.

✔ The stethoscope includes an acceptable length of tubing between the bell and the earpieces. Tubing that's too long may diminish the sound so that it can't be heard.

To ensure an accurate reading when using a mercury blood pressure gauge, make sure that

✔ The top of the column of mercury registers at zero with no air pressure in the blood pressure gauge.

✔ The column of mercury is vertical.

✔ The tubing is clean and unobstructed. If you disconnect the tubing, you should be able to blow air through it. If air doesn't flow freely through the tubing, get new tubing.

✔ The size of the cuff *(bladder)* is correct.

• A cuff that's too narrow for the patient's arm gives a high reading.

• A cuff that's too wide for the patient's arm gives a low reading.

Sidestepping faulty observation and patient problems

To avoid faulty observation, make sure that

✔ The person taking your blood pressure doesn't allow a preconceived notion of how high or low your blood pressure may be to influence the reading.

✔ The person who measures your blood pressure writes down your reading instead of memorizing it. Poor memory often leads to an inaccurate charting of the numbers.

To avoid patient problems and ensure an accurate blood pressure reading, make sure

> ✔ The patient's arm is at heart level. If the arm is above heart level, the reading may be inaccurately high. If the arm is below heart level, the reading may be inaccurately low.
>
> ✔ The patient's back is supported and the patient's legs aren't dangling.
>
> ✔ That if the patient has a large, muscular arm (that may cause an inaccurately high reading), a blood pressure gauge that has a cuff that's large enough to accommodate is used.
>
> ✔ That if the patient has calcified arteries (common among the elderly) that are hard to compress, another method of blood pressure measurement such as direct insertion of a blood pressure gauge into the artery is used.

Whew! There are quite a few things to keep in mind while taking your blood pressure. After you have an accurate reading, it's time to process the numbers. Read on for more about what the numbers mean.

Comprehending the Numbers

When your doctor says, "Your blood pressure is 135 over 85," for example, what do the numbers really mean?

The first number is the *systolic blood pressure* (SBP) — the amount of pressure in your arteries as the heart pumps. *Systole* is the rhythmic contraction of your heart muscle when it's expelling blood from your left ventricle — the large chamber on the left side of your heart. The aortic valve sits between that chamber and your *aorta,* the large artery that takes blood away from the heart to the rest of the body. During systole, the aortic valve is open and blood flows freely to the rest of your body.

The second number is the *diastolic blood pressure* (DBP). After your heart empties the blood from the ventricle, the aortic valve shuts to prevent blood from returning into the heart from the rest of your body. Your heart muscle relaxes and the ventricle expands as blood fills it up from the left atrium, which has received it from the lungs. Within your arteries, the blood pressure rapidly falls until it reaches its lowest point. The diastolic blood pressure — the second number that's read on the gauge or the top of the mercury column reflects this lowest point of blood pressure. Before it falls further, the ventricle contracts again and the blood pressure starts to rise back up to the systolic level.

After you've established your SBP and DBP, determine whether your blood pressure is high and whether it should be treated. But first, how high is too high?

At birth, your blood pressure is around 90/60 mm Hg or even lower. As you grow older, it gradually rises until as an adult your blood pressure is generally between 120/80 mm Hg and 139/89 mm Hg. Higher than that and you're considered to have high blood pressure.

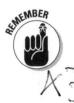

No fixed number serves as a guide for your diastolic or systolic blood pressure that tells you your blood pressure is high if it's above the number or low if it's below the number. Doctors established 140/90 mm Hg as the point at which action is taken, but the fact remains that a person with a blood pressure reading of 120/80 mm Hg is at lower risk of blood pressure complications than a person with a 130/85 mm Hg.

The National Heart, Lung, and Blood Institute, a division of the National Institutes of Health, established the Joint National Committee on Prevention, Detection, Evaluation, and Treatment of High Blood Pressure. The committee created a Classification of Blood Pressure for Adults that's shown in Table 2-1. Use the table to determine whether your blood pressure measurement is normal or abnormal. If your blood pressure falls in the high-normal or high blood pressure categories, discuss treatment with your doctor. (Refer to Part III for information on successful treatment options.) *Note:* When SBP and DBP fall into different categories, use the higher category. Also, Hg is the chemical notation for mercury.

Table 2-1	Classification of Blood Pressure for Adults*		
Category	*SBP (mm Hg)*		*DBP (mm Hg)*
Optimal	<120	and	<80
Normal	<130	and	<85
High-normal	130–139	or	85–89
Stage 1 HBP	140–159	or	90–99
Stage 2 HBP	160–179	or	100–109
Stage 3 HBP	180+	or	110+

*As noted by the Joint National Committee on Prevention, Detection, Evaluation, and Treatment of High Blood Pressure.

Can Blood Pressure Be Too Low?

Blood pressure can certainly be too low in a number of situations, especially if too much blood-pressure-lowering medication is taken. People can tolerate many different levels of blood pressure without symptoms. If the pressure is too low, however, the patient becomes dizzy upon standing, when too much blood pools in the legs. Then some kind of treatment is needed to raise the blood pressure. This happens particularly in diabetic patients. Other situations where the blood pressure may be too low include prolonged bed rest and bleeding or dehydration. Such patients discover how to get up slowly to give the body a chance to adjust.

Recognizing Variable Pressure Readings

Blood pressure varies widely. If you check the blood pressure of a group of people at many different times of day or night, you'll find some amazing variations. For example, one person's blood pressure during the day can vary from 175/100 mm Hg, a high blood pressure, to 105/60 mm Hg, a healthy, normal blood pressure. Some of the reasons for the variability are

- ✔ Blood pressure tends to drop during sleep

- ✔ Blood pressure quickly increases when you awaken

- ✔ Respiration and heart rate affect blood pressure

- ✔ Mental and physical activity affect blood pressure

- ✔ The nighttime fall in blood pressure is less in the elderly or people with diabetes

- ✔ Smoking raises blood pressure with each cigarette

- ✔ Sleep deprivation raises blood pressure

- ✔ Defecation or a bladder full of urine may raise blood pressure

- ✔ Consuming more than two ounces of alcohol on a daily basis raises blood pressure

Another factor that often causes a rise in blood pressure is the *white coat effect.* Something about physicians frightens patients because, when experiencing the white coat effect, your systolic blood pressure may be ten millimeters of mercury higher when taken by a physician as compared to when the nurse takes it. Even the nurse can have a mild white coat effect; if you take your blood pressure at home, it may be five millimeters or so lower than the nurse's reading.

Experiencing the white coat effect does not mean, however, that you're okay if your blood pressure is normal at home but not in the doctor's office. All the studies that show improvement in the rates of stroke, heart attacks, and other complications are based on measurements made in the doctor's office. People with white-coat high blood pressure seem to be different from the population with normal blood pressure because those with white-coat high blood pressure also have other associated health problems, such as high blood glucose and cholesterol. Thus their high blood pressure most probably represents an abnormality consistent with their other abnormalities.

Taking Your Blood Pressure at Home

Often patients who register a high reading in the doctor's office register a normal reading at home. While normal home measurements don't mean that you can avoid treatment if your blood pressure is high in the doctor's office, a number of advantages exist to measuring your own blood pressure at home. First, you can identify whether you have white-coat high blood pressure. (Refer to the "Recognizing Variable Pressure Readings" section, earlier in this chapter, for more on white-coat high blood pressure.) More importantly, frequent measurements of your blood pressure can tell you whether your treatment is working. More readings can overcome the problem of your blood pressure variability.

Home readings of your blood pressure can also make you adhere to the treatment because you get rapid feedback. You know whether the diet, exercise, or pills are working, and you'll be able to alter the treatment long before your next office visit by getting in touch with your doctor by phone or e-mail. You may reduce the cost of care because you won't have to see your doctor as often if your blood pressure remains stable and low.

Because the home pressure tends to be lower, a normal pressure at home is considered to be less than 135/85 mm Hg.

Numerous devices are on the market for monitoring blood pressure at home. Some use the wrist or finger as the site of the blood pressure measurement, but I don't recommend them because they tend to be inaccurate with rare exceptions. I also don't recommend using a mercury blood pressure gauge at home. Other types of blood pressure gauges are just as accurate and avoid the risk of mercury contamination.

The best home devices are electronic devices that measure the blood pressure at the elbow and don't require you to do anything more than attach the cuff properly and press a button to turn it on. The device then inflates the cuff, measures the blood pressure, and gives a reading on a screen. After checking numerous articles comparing these devices, the Omron HEM-737AC is highly accurate, reliable, and should cost around $100, which is a small price to pay for this level of quality.

Even if you purchase one of these highly reliable home blood pressure monitoring devices, you must compare it with the results obtained on a mercury blood pressure gauge at least once a year (every six months is even better) in your doctor's office. Accuracy is critical.

Taking an Ambulatory Reading

An ambulatory reading is done using a portable device called an *ambulatory blood pressure monitor*. It consists of a cuff attached to your arm and to a machine that pumps up the cuff and measures the blood pressure every 15 to 30 minutes during the day and every 30 to 60 minutes at night. Of course, the device is visible. The machine records the results and displays them when downloaded into a computer.

Your doctor may want to check your blood pressure many times during one 24-hour period for a variety of reasons, such as to

- Assess white-coat high blood pressure
- Determine if and the reason you're resistant to drugs
- Check on low blood pressure symptoms
- Evaluate sporadic high blood pressure

Interestingly, ambulatory blood pressure monitors show that up to 30 percent of high office blood pressures are due to the white coat effect.

Getting the Right Post-Diagnosis

If, by chance, you're unable to prevent yourself from developing high blood pressure, you want to make sure that your doctor evaluates your blood pressure properly. Assuming this is a first visit to the doctor for established high blood pressure, the doctor must make a number of assessments that can be categorized as history, physical examination, and lab testing.

Assessing your history

Your history describes your past association with high blood pressure. It's similar to a history taken for any other condition with a few variations specific to high blood pressure. The important points in the history are

- Duration of high blood pressure (when it was first discovered)
- Course of the blood pressure (whether it has always been high since it was discovered)
- Treatment with drugs, diet, exercise, or other means

- Use of agents that could worsen blood pressure, such as steroids, birth control pills, and nonsteroidal anti-inflammatory agents

- Any family history of high blood pressure

- Symptoms that may suggest secondary high blood pressure (see Chapter 4)

- Symptoms of the consequences of high blood pressure (see Part II)

- Presence of other risk factors, such as smoking, diabetes, and high cholesterol

- Social factors, such as family structure, work, and education

- Dietary history

- Sexual function (to evaluate before using drugs that affect it)

- Possibility of sleep apnea (a condition in which an individual gasps for breath and snores during sleep following several stops in breathing)

Evaluating your physical exam

After the doctor notes the history, a physical examination should be done. This is also mostly a routine evaluation with some special studies because of the high blood pressure. The main parts of the exam are

- Abdominal exam to look for tumors or abnormal sounds suggesting restricted blood flow

- Blood pressure reading as described earlier in this chapter

- Body fat distribution

- Examination of the neck for thyroid or blood vessel abnormalities

- Examination of the pulses in the arteries

- Heart exam

- Internal eye exam

- Lung exam

- Neurological exam

Sending samples to the lab

Your history and physical exam can give the doctor an excellent idea of the severity of the problem and the possibility that secondary high blood pressure is present. Then lab tests are used to get a general picture of your overall health and to look for specific abnormalities that the history and physical pointed to. The key lab tests done on everyone with high blood pressure are

- Complete blood count
- Serum chemistry profile that looks at the sodium, potassium, liver function, and the kidney function.
- Lipid profile that evaluates cholesterol and triglycerides
- Microalbumin test to look for early kidney disease

If definite damage associated with high blood pressure is suspected, the doctor should do other studies. For example:

- **Brain abnormalities:** The doctor might do a study called a Doppler flow study to check for blockage of blood vessels in the neck.
- **Heart disease:** Do an electrocardiogram and chest X-ray.
- **Kidney problems:** Check for increased uric acid using a blood test.

In Chapter 4, you can find the specific tests to be done if secondary high blood pressure is suspected. Key elements in the history and physical that may lead a doctor to do these tests are the sudden onset of high blood pressure, especially under the age of 20 or above the age of 50 and blood pressure that's especially elevated. A low potassium level or a poor response to treatment also suggests a secondary cause of the high blood pressure.

You can use these preceding guidelines to determine whether your doctor is doing everything that should be done to evaluate your high blood pressure. You may find something that's been left out. Don't hesitate to inform the doctor and get the study. It's a matter of your health and your life.

Chapter 3

Determining If You Are At Risk

Many factors play a role in the development of high blood pressure. Some factors, such as your family history, ethnic background, age, and gender, can't be controlled while other factors, such as diet, exercise, stress, your smoking and drinking habits, and a tendency to park as close to the exercise facility as possible, can be controlled. Each factor may be present to a greater or lesser extent in a particular area of the world, so that in some places the prevalence of high blood pressure is low while in others the prevalence of high blood pressure is extremely high and the consequences (see Part II) are severe.

In this chapter, I discuss both the uncontrollable and the controllable factors related to the development of high blood pressure. If you haven't been diagnosed with high blood pressure, be sure to read up on the controllable factors that, if managed over time, can help lessen your chances of developing high blood pressure. If you've been diagnosed with high blood pressure, be sure to read Part III where I discuss the same controllable factors in relation to treating high blood pressure.

One of the factors that may cause your blood pressure to rise is forgetting your spouse's birthday. Running over the kid's bicycle as you back into the garage may also cause a rise in blood pressure. So be real careful as you're backing your car into the garage. However, if you should forget a loved one's birthday or back over your son's bike, your blood pressure will only rise temporarily.

Factoring in What You Can't Control

This section describes the factors in your life that you can't control. Your family history, ethnic background, gender, and age can't be altered. These uncontrollable factors aren't quite the same as the problem that arises when you hang something in your closet for a while, and it shrinks two sizes.

Although you can't control these factors, knowing how they contribute to high blood pressure is important. However, don't think that you don't have to be cautious. Allow yourself to become obese, and you may be the exception who has high blood pressure in your group.

Looking at the global picture

The prevalence of high blood pressure throughout the world can be broken down into four major categories as follows:

- **Zero:** A few isolated groups, such as in the Amazon, have zero high blood pressure.

- **Low:** The incidence of high blood pressure is low (below 15 percent) in the rural populations of Latin and South America, China, and Africa.

- **Normal:** Most often, high blood pressure prevails in about 15 to 30 percent of a given population, such as in most of the industrialized nations — Japan, Europe, and the Caucasian population of the United States.

- **High:** A high percentage (30 to 40 percent) is found in the Russian Federation, Finland, Poland, and among African Americans.

Wherever high blood pressure is found, heart, brain, and kidney complications are similarly high. The burden of disease due to high blood pressure is enormous in countries like the Russian Federation but no more than among African Americans. (See the "African Americans" section later in this chapter.) Brain attack, usually related to high blood pressure, is the second leading cause of death in Japan, and a continued emphasis on blood pressure control to prevent stroke is the way to go per a study in *Stroke* (August 2001).

Several studies conducted throughout the world on high blood pressure show that a high percentage of high blood pressure in various populations often coexists with poor awareness and insufficient treatment. For example, a study in the *Archives of Brazilian Cardiology* (July 2001) shows that the percentages of high blood pressure in Brazil are similar to the United States, but only a fraction of the population with high blood pressure in Brazil can control it. And similarly, several European populations were aware of their high blood pressure but unable to control it. For example, in Spain they use a blood pressure of 160/95 mm Hg as the cutoff point to begin treatment rather than 140/90 mm Hg while in France both awareness and treatment are inadequate. The blood pressure of many South Koreans is also generally on the high end. And although many receive treatment, few South Koreans are able to control their high blood pressure per a study in the *Journal of Hypertension* (September 2001).

The Stroke Belt

The Stroke Belt includes most of the southeastern United States with the exception of Florida. The greater prevalence of high blood pressure in the southeastern United States means that large numbers of strokes (brain attacks) occur there. In fact, deaths due to brain attacks in the southeastern United States number more than 10 percent above the national average. But brain attacks aren't the only consequence of high blood pressure. Other complications due to high blood pressure, such as kidney failure and heart failure, occur far more often in the Southeast than the rest of the country. (For more on kidney failure and heart failure, see Part II.) The overall death rate is higher in the southeastern states as compared to the rest of the country.

Caucasian men have a somewhat higher prevalence of high blood pressure in the Southeast as compared to the rest of the country. Low birth weight along with high blood pressure is also more frequent among African Americans in the Southeast, the area of the country where most African Americans live.

However, the reasons that African Americans in the southeastern United States have such high rates of high blood pressure and death due to its complications are no different from the reasons for high blood pressure in general:

- ✔ **High salt intake** is common in the Southeast, especially among African Americans.

- ✔ **Low potassium intake** from fruits and vegetables is usual.

- ✔ **Obesity** is greatly increased.

- ✔ **Physical inactivity** is the rule in the Southeast. Half of the population doesn't get enough exercise.

Before you pack your bags and fly off to the Amazon, however, in the hopes of living a long, illness-free retirement in a tropical Paradise, please consider that if a high percentage of high blood pressure often coexists with poor awareness and insufficient treatment, then perhaps low percentages can coexist with acute awareness and sufficient treatment. Read on.

Accounting for the contribution of your genes

High blood pressure tends to run in families. A family history of high blood pressure can predict the development of high blood pressure in relatives with normal blood pressure. So if you have two or more relatives who developed high blood pressure before the age of 55, you're at much higher risk of developing it yourself. Next time around, try to pick your parents a little more carefully.

For example, when adopted children were compared with biological children, the same or similar blood pressure measurements were shared between biological parents and children than between adopted children and parents.

Heredity also affects body weight. People who are closely related tend to have similar degrees of obesity, which plays a large role in the development of high blood pressure. (See the "Exercising and controlling your weight" section later in this chapter.)

The *insulin resistance syndrome* may be a particularly important example of the role that inheritance plays in high blood pressure. People with this condition have increased *insulin* (the hormone that controls blood sugar) with reduced sensitivity to their insulin. They show a typical pattern of blood fats consisting of high triglycerides (the type of fat found on meat — greater than 200 mg/dL) and low HDL cholesterol (the blood fat particle that protects against heart attacks — less than 30 mg/dL). They're usually but not always obese. People who suffer from insulin resistance syndrome tend to have a much higher incidence of fatal heart attacks and may make up 20 percent of all high blood pressure cases. Their fat tends to be around the waistline.

Estimating the effects of ethnicity

According to the U.S. Centers for Disease Control, the prevalence of high blood pressure was reduced among men and women in every ethnic group between 1960 and 1990. Some representative differences are shown in Table 3-1.

Table 3-1	Percentage of U.S. Population Age 20 and Older with High Blood Pressure*			
Group	*1960*	*1970*	*1980*	*1990*
Both sexes	36.9	38.3	39.0	23.1
Male	40.0	42.4	44.0	25.3
Female	33.7	34.4	34.0	20.8
Caucasian Male	39.3	41.7	43.5	24.3
Caucasian Female	31.7	32.4	32.3	19.3
African American Male	48.1	51.8	48.7	34.9
African American Female	50.8	50.3	47.5	33.8
Hispanic Male			25.0	25.2
Hispanic Female			21.8	22.0

Percentages provided by the U.S. Centers for Disease Control.

The table shows the great strides that have been made to reduce the prevalence of high blood pressure in this 30-year period but still indicates that a quarter of the age-20-and-older population suffers from high blood pressure and one out of three African Americans has high blood pressure. When coupled with appropriate medical attention and lifestyle changes, an awareness of these factors can lower the number of high blood pressure cases around the world.

Salt
√Fat
Low Potassium
Low Activity

African Americans

African Americans — the population most at-risk in the United States of developing high blood pressure and its consequences — develop high blood pressure twice as often as Caucasians. African Americans also have a high rate of kidney failure, called *end-stage renal disease,* and this may be due in part to their increased level of high blood pressure. African Americans may have an inherited kidney defect that limits their ability to handle salt. African Americans also have less response to nitric oxide than Caucasians. (For more on nitric oxide, see Chapter 1 and the "Nitric oxide" sidebar in this chapter.) In addition, the stresses of living associated with low socioeconomic status are frequently blamed for at least some of the high blood pressure among African Americans.

Identifying the culprits: Salt and fat *low Potassium (fruits veg)*

Comparing people of the same race in different areas of the world, a study in *Scientific American* in February 1999 sought an explanation for the high rate of high blood pressure among African Americans. The authors, dissatisfied with a genetic explanation, found great differences between Africans living in Nigeria, Jamaica, and the United States:

✔ Nigerians are generally lean, do physically demanding work, and eat a traditional Nigerian diet of rice, vegetables, and fruits. Blood pressure doesn't rise as they get older, and high blood pressure is rare.

✔ The Jamaican diet is a mixture of food that Jamaicans grow themselves and commercial food. They tend to live six years longer than African Americans because the incidence of cancer and heart disease is lower.

✔ An African American community living outside of Chicago in Maywood, which is made up of migrants from the Southeastern United States, has a high-salt, high-fat diet.

✔ Although all the groups studied had a common genetic background, the percentage of the population with high blood pressure was 7 percent for the Nigerians, 26 percent for the Jamaicans, and 33 percent for the African Americans, who have the greater body weight, greater salt intake, and less potassium intake than Africans in Africa.

The authors concluded that no racial explanation exists — high blood pressure in African Americans isn't genetic because African Americans with high blood pressure and those with normal blood pressure share the same genes. Explanations for differences in this abnormality should be sought in the environment and not in the genes.

Dietary treatment, however, has been particularly successful among African Americans with high blood pressure. One of the best approaches has been the DASH diet, the Dietary Approach to Stop Hypertension (see Chapter 9), consisting of increased amounts of fruits and vegetables and grains, low-fat dairy products, and protein low in total and saturated fats.

Hispanics

Compared to other ethnic groups in the United States, the prevalence of high blood pressure among Hispanics is generally similar to Caucasians. Although the incidence of high blood pressure is greater among African Americans than Hispanics, Hispanic adults tend not to take medication for their high blood pressure as often as Caucasians or African Americans.

Caucasians

About 25 percent of adult Caucasians in the United States have high blood pressure. Caucasians, as a group, seem to be more aware of their high blood pressure and get treatment more often than African Americans or Hispanics. However, treatment is satisfactory only around 20 percent of the time, so there is much room for improvement in this group as well.

Focusing on gender

In young adults, high blood pressure is more prevalent in men than women. But after women reach the age of 50 (when most women lose their estrogen through menopause or removal of their ovaries), women have a higher prevalence of high blood pressure than men.

More often than men, women tend to be aware of their high blood pressure, get treatment for it, and control it. This may be because women see doctors more frequently for pregnancies, pelvic exams, and breast exams, and the high blood pressure is noted at those visits.

Similar to men, women reduce their risk of brain attack when treated for high blood pressure, so treatment should be given to women just as often as it's given to men.

Going past menopause

Postmenopausal women, even those who have normal blood pressure, respond to stress in such a way as to raise their blood pressure as compared to women who have not yet reached menopause. The estrogen loss that occurs during menopause may not just be the only factor; the weight gain that accompanies aging and other factors may also contribute to the rise in blood pressure.

Postmenopausal women are actually more sensitive to salt than men. This may be an additional reason for their increased tendency towards high blood pressure.

Taking estrogenic hormones doesn't seem to elevate blood pressure or make the postmenopausal woman more sensitive to salt or stress. Postmenopausal women who have high blood pressure may be given estrogens because their blood pressure isn't made worse.

Taking oral contraceptives

Previously, oral contraceptives contained more estrogen and progesterone and their use was associated with more heart disease, heart attacks, brain attacks, and a higher death rate. Current preparations contain less hormone and are much safer, especially in comparison to other methods of contraception. Oral contraceptives can cause a slight increase in blood clots and in breast cancer, however; so oral contraceptives shouldn't be given to a woman who has had blood clots in the past.

Oral contraceptives are associated with some rise in blood pressure that subsides when use is discontinued. Once in a while, oral contraceptives can bring on more severe high blood pressure. If a patient has a family history of high blood pressure or kidney disease, oral contraceptives need to be given with care and blood pressure needs to be monitored frequently.

Exactly why blood pressure rises as a result of taking oral contraceptives is unclear. High blood pressure associated with oral contraceptives may be due to the amount of progesterone rather than estrogen in the preparation. Those preparations that have less progesterone or intermittent progesterone are less often connected to high blood pressure in the patient.

If the blood pressure doesn't return to normal when the oral contraceptive is discontinued, the woman should be evaluated for some other cause for her high blood pressure. If no other form of contraception can be used, combining the oral contraceptive with a blood-pressure-lowering drug may be necessary. (See Chapter 13 for more information on pressure-lowering medications.)

Rising in stages with age

Blood pressure tends to go up with age for many reasons — loss of kidney function, less ability to rid the body of salt, hardening of the arteries, increasing obesity, and greater sensitivity to the blood-pressure-raising effect of even more normal levels of salt.

With aging, the blood pressure tends to rise in stages. Although these stages are variable for some individuals, high blood pressure usually develops in a fairly orderly fashion from pre-high blood pressure to sustained high blood pressure.

High blood pressure can occur before age thirty, but the following discussion presents the usual sequence of events. Between birth and the age of thirty, the pre-high blood pressure stage, occasional blood pressure measurements may be high, but the elevation isn't constant. This is a clue that high blood pressure will develop. Other clues include some of the following:

- Birth weight is low.
- Blood pressure rises excessively during stress or exercise.
- Random pressures are high/normal (close to 140/90 mm Hg).
- Other features, such as obesity, increased alcohol intake, diabetes, reduced HDL, or increased triglycerides, may be present.

The next stage may last five to ten years but is usually found between the ages of 30 to 40. In this stage, high blood pressure is often found, but periods of normal blood pressure follow.

The stage of sustained high blood pressure may begin as early as 30 years of age, but *essential hypertension* (high blood pressure for which the cause cannot be determined) usually occurs by the age of 50. People who suffer from essential hypertension at age 50 or sooner are highly susceptible to early heart attacks and brain attacks. If left untreated, their life expectancy is reduced 15 to 20 years.

If high blood pressure develops past the age of 50, it's more likely to be secondary high blood pressure, as explained in Chapter 4. Chapter 14 discusses the problems of blood pressure in the elderly at greater length.

Working on Factors Within Your Control

In the United States, two million new patients are diagnosed with high blood pressure every year. Although you can't change the genes that you received from your parents, you can change many lifestyle behaviors to prevent high blood pressure. For starters, as an adult, you should be screened for high blood pressure at least every two years. Other changes you can make include

- Reducing your stress using humor (see Chapter 8)
- Increasing your potassium intake by eating more fruits and vegetables (see Chapter 9)
- Reducing daily salt intake to less than 6,000 milligrams (1 teaspoon), which is equal to 2,400 milligrams of salt (see Chapter 10)
- Keeping alcohol intake to two drinks or less per day (see Chapter 11)
- Controlling your weight through diet and exercise (see Chapter 12)

All the techniques that you use to prevent high blood pressure can work to lower blood pressure after it's present. The great difference between using these techniques to prevent high blood pressure as compared to treating established high blood pressure is the cost and the risks associated with taking medication that will almost certainly be needed. That's why it's important to remember: If you can prevent high blood pressure, do everything in your power to do so. You won't be sorry.

Taking it with a grain of salt

The typical diet throughout the wealthier nations of the world contains too much salt. Evidence abounds that this is so. Not all people, however, develop high blood pressure; only about half the population. Those who have high blood pressure must have some form of increased sensitivity. (The same amount of salt raises their blood pressure to a greater extent.) The evidence for the role of salt comes from studies of populations as well as experimental manipulation of salt intake to raise and lower blood pressure. The population studies noted that

- Primitive tribes that don't eat salt have zero high blood pressure, and they don't have the consequences of high blood pressure, such as damage to the heart, kidney, or brain.
- These same primitive people given salt develop high blood pressure and its consequences.
- The more salt that's consumed, the higher the blood pressure.

In terms of interventions, studies concluded that

- When people with high blood pressure are salt-restricted, they lower their blood pressure.
- Babies who are given a low-salt diet have lower blood pressures.
- Animals given more salt show a rise in blood pressure.

This sensitivity to salt seems to be inherited from the mother because she usually has the same rise in blood pressure after eating salt as her offspring. A person without salt sensitivity excretes most of an excess salt intake along with water in the kidneys, but a person with salt sensitivity can't do this as easily. See Chapter 10 for more information on salt intake.

Blood pressure, however, doesn't always fall when salt is restricted because some people respond to salt in a different manner than others. Certain groups are more salt sensitive. These include

- Diabetics
- Older individuals

✔ People whose kidneys are failing

✔ People who don't produce enough of an enzyme that raises blood pressure called *renin* in their kidneys

Lowering your salt intake can help reduce your chances of developing high blood pressure. Paying attention to product labels and choosing foods labeled "sodium-free" or "reduced-sodium" is one way to monitor your salt intake. I detail other practical ways to reduce your salt intake in Chapter 10.

Chilling out

Essential high blood pressure (high blood pressure for which the cause is unknown) is about half due to inheritance and half due to the environment. The major factors in the environment are diet and psychological and social stresses.

Many groups show the difference between the development of high blood pressure in stressful situations as compared to low stress environments. For example:

✔ A study in the *New England Journal of Medicine* (March 1968) of several nuns isolated in Italy as compared to a group of women in regular society showed that although blood pressures were the same at the beginning, after 30 years, the nuns had blood pressures 30 millimeters lower than the controls.

✔ People who go from "low-stress" societies to "higher-stress" societies show sustained increases in blood pressure.

✔ People who work in jobs where they have little control but much responsibility also show elevated blood pressures.

✔ Air traffic controllers have higher blood pressures as a group than less stressful occupations.

✔ African Americans growing up in higher stress environments have a higher incidence of high blood pressure.

Some of these studies have been questioned because other factors may be playing a role. For example, the diet of the nuns may have been less likely to cause high blood pressure, especially when eaten over 30 years. People going to "higher stress" societies are also eating more salt than they did before.

Some studies show a correlation between internalized anger and others don't. Whether blood pressure tends to be high in certain individuals who turn their anger inward instead of responding by an external show of anger or some other external act, such as increased exercise, is still the subject of much controversy.

Finally, whether people who respond to stress by reacting excessively tend to develop high blood pressure more often than those who are less reactive is unknown. Studies of this phenomenon are again inconsistent.

While many studies on stress and high blood pressure result in inconsistent findings, one thing is for sure: Reducing the level of stress in your life can only be a good thing. The less stressed you are, the less likely you are to overeat, smoke, and drink excessively — all factors that are known to cause high blood pressure.

Exercising and controlling your weight

The significance of an inactive lifestyle in the development of high blood pressure is clear. In study after study, those who exercise more have a lower incidence of high blood pressure. An active lifestyle promotes weight control.

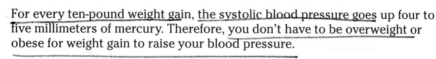

For every ten-pound weight gain, the systolic blood pressure goes up four to five millimeters of mercury. Therefore, you don't have to be overweight or obese for weight gain to raise your blood pressure.

Central obesity (fat in the waist area) is associated with high blood pressure more than obesity in the legs and thighs. A large waistline is a good clue that high blood pressure is on its way or has already arrived.

The insulin resistance syndrome, described earlier in this chapter in the "Accounting for the contribution of your genes" section, is a condition that contains factors that combine to place the patient at high risk of heart disease. Those factors include obesity, high blood pressure, elevated levels of insulin and insulin resistance, central distribution of fat, high triglycerides, low HDL ("good" cholesterol), higher levels of LDL ("bad" cholesterol), high levels of uric acid in the bloodstream, type 2 diabetes mellitus, and high levels of chemicals that prevent clots from breaking down, all of which predispose patients to heart attacks.

Just how obesity results in higher blood pressure is unclear. People who are obese have increased cardiac output and increased peripheral resistance; more blood needs to be pumped to provide nutrients to their increased tissues. But many organs, particularly the kidneys, don't accept increased blood flow and produce hormones to reduce it by narrowing the arteries, thus increasing peripheral resistance and blood pressure. Obese people often take in more salt than lean people, and they're more sensitive to the blood pressure raising effect of the salt. Obesity is also associated with an increase in the activity of the nervous system, which can cause narrowing of blood vessels.

In Chapter 9, you'll find recommendations for weight loss as one treatment of high blood pressure. Combined with exercise and salt and alcohol reduction, weight loss can have a profound blood-pressure-lowering effect. These measures should always precede pressure-lowering medications unless the blood pressure is dangerously high (greater than 180/120 mm Hg). Part of the positive effects of these lifestyle changes may be through improvement in the insulin resistance syndrome leading to reduced insulin and its role in raising blood pressure.

Of course, you don't want to take this exercise program too far. My grandmother started walking five miles a day at age 60. She's 97 now, and nobody knows where the heck she is.

Smoking and excessive drinking

Using tobacco in any form and drinking excessively (see Chapter 11) have been shown to raise blood pressure while the absence of smoking and drinking lowers blood pressure. Tobacco and alcohol cause all kinds of other problems for you, too, but their effect on your blood pressure is enough reason to stop using them.

The various factors mentioned in this chapter that lead to high blood pressure is far from inclusive. I stress the most important factors, but scientists are discovering other factors that cause high blood pressure on an almost daily basis. If you want to discover more about the latest research, check out Chapter 20 and go to one of the references found there.

Nitric oxide

The cells that line the inside of the blood vessels produce nitric oxide. Nitric oxide is a potent compound that widens blood vessels and reduces blood pressure. A number of so-called "risk factors for cardiovascular disease" pose an increased risk to the heart, precipitate strokes, and cause damage to the cells that line the inside of the blood vessels and inhibit their ability to produce nitric oxide; these risk factors include

✔ High blood pressure

✔ High cholesterol

✔ Insulin resistance

✔ The postmenopausal lack of estrogen

✔ Tobacco smoking or chewing

Reversing any of these risk factors eliminates their damaging effects to the blood vessels and their contribution to the inhibition of nitric oxide production inside the blood vessels. When these risk factors are present, however, they also make the individual more susceptible to the blood-pressure-raising effect of stress. The way to attack any of these risk factors can be found in Part III.

Education would go a long way toward helping these and other poorly controlled high blood pressure patients get their blood pressure under control and avoid the brain attacks and heart attacks that are otherwise inevitable. Just like the studies on other countries, a high percentage of high blood pressure often coexists with poor awareness and insufficient treatment.

Chapter 4

Understanding Secondary High Blood Pressure

- -

In This Chapter

▶ Discovering secondary high blood pressure early on

▶ Dealing with renal vascular high blood pressure

▶ Finding a tumor that induces secondary high blood pressure

▶ Regulating an overabundance of cortisol

▶ Coping with causes that you're born with and more

- -

*T*his chapter introduces you to a few multisyllabic medical terms — real tongue twisters, such as *pheochromocytoma* — the names of tumors, diseases, and disorders that can bring on some unhealthy symptoms, such as secondary high blood pressure. While you read my descriptions, you may imagine that you indeed have the disease. But chances are, you're more likely to win the lottery or be hit by a bolt of lightning than contract any one of these rare diseases. Of course, if you get one of these diseases, you'll be the only one on your block. I recommend that you express your uniqueness some other way.

The upside of secondary high blood pressure is that after the disease that's causing it is identified and treated, you're like new most of the time. The high blood pressure and the other signs and symptoms of the disease disappear. Your whole life will improve — even your piano playing (if you then take lessons).

So before you let your imagination run wild, ask your doctor. If your doctor's opinion doesn't satisfy you, then get a second opinion from another physician.

Secondary high blood pressure means that a specific disease causes the high blood pressure — the high blood pressure is one of several signs and symptoms associated with the disease. If the person is cured of the disease that's causing the secondary high blood pressure, then the high blood pressure is lowered. Treatment of the disease often eliminates the high blood pressure.

Although secondary high blood pressure makes up only 5 percent of the total number of high blood pressure cases, its causes are important. A careful history, physical exam, and lab evaluation (as discussed in Chapter 2) can help a physician discover the disease that's causing your blood pressure to rise. This chapter introduces you to some of the most common causes of secondary high blood pressure, how the diagnosis is confirmed in each case, and the appropriate treatment.

It's important that I emphasize that treating the disease or disorder that's causing the secondary high blood pressure can lower your blood pressure, but lifestyle changes can also lower secondary high blood pressure independent of the disease or disorder. Thus weight loss (see Chapter 9), exercise (see Chapter 12), stopping smoking (see Chapter 11), and reducing salt in your diet (see Chapter 10) can make a big difference.

Nipping Secondary High Blood Pressure in the Bud

Several clues that should prompt an investigation for secondary high blood pressure include

- ✔ Damage to the eyes, kidneys, or heart
- ✔ Family history of kidney disease
- ✔ Flushing spells when your skin turns red and hot
- ✔ Increased body pigmentation and pigmented stretch marks
- ✔ Intolerance to heat
- ✔ Loud humming sound in the abdomen (called a *bruit*)
- ✔ Low potassium level in the blood
- ✔ Poor response to usually effective treatment for high blood pressure
- ✔ Rapid pulse
- ✔ The onset of high blood pressure before age 20 or past age 50
- ✔ Unusually high level of high blood pressure (above 180/120 mm Hg)

If you notice any of these in the preceding list, point it out to your doctor. By finding and treating secondary high blood pressure early, you're more certain to have a return to normal blood pressure before permanent changes occur. Some changes, such as kidney damage, can affect your high blood pressure permanently even if the disease or disorder that's causing the secondary high blood pressure is eliminated.

Secondary High Blood Pressure and Your Kidneys

At some point or other, the kidneys get involved when high blood pressure is present. Damage to the kidneys may precede the high blood pressure. Then the high blood pressure is secondary. If the high blood pressure precedes the kidney damage, the high blood pressure is primary or *essential*. Two main conditions of the kidney, damaged kidney tissue and blocked kidney arteries, can lead to high blood pressure.

Discovering damaged kidney tissue

Damaged kidney tissue is the most common reason for secondary high blood pressure, accounting for about 50 percent of the cases. *Renal* (kidney) *parenchymal* (tissue) *hypertension* (high blood pressure) results from a kidney-damaging illness, such as diabetes, use of certain medications, an inflammation of the kidney, or a hereditary disease that results in *cysts* (sacs filled with fluid). The damaged kidneys don't function normally and can't eliminate sodium at a normal rate, resulting in salt and water retention that leads to high blood pressure.

Diagnosing chronic and acute kidney tissue loss

Loss of kidney tissue that leads to high blood pressure can be *chronic* (slow to develop) or *acute* (sudden). Some of the diseases and conditions that cause chronic kidney damage are

 ✔ Chronic obstruction of the *ureter* (the tube that takes urine from the kidney to the bladder)

 ✔ Cysts that displace normal kidney tissue

 ✔ Damage to the *glomerulus* (the filtering part of the kidney)

 ✔ Diabetes mellitus (diabetic kidney disease)

The details of diabetic kidney disease

Diabetes mellitus, a particularly damaging disease that may affect the kidneys, is the most common cause of kidney damage and kidney failure. It usually takes 15 or more years of poorly controlled diabetes to reach the point of affecting the kidneys. Most people that have diabetes mellitus also have high blood pressure as well as the characteristic eye disease seen in diabetes called *diabetic retinopathy.* Certain drugs called *ACE inhibitors* (see Chapter 13) are particularly helpful in slowing the progression of diabetic kidney disease and may even reverse it.

In diabetic kidney disease, the most important treatments consist of controlling blood glucose (sugar), blood pressure, and blood cholesterol. Diabetics should restrict their salt intake as well as their protein, which seems to make the kidney disease worse.

Controlling the secondary high blood pressure present in all the conditions in this preceding list is important because continued high blood pressure acting on the kidneys can damage the kidneys further and lead to even higher blood pressure. It's a vicious cycle.

High blood pressure also accompanies acute kidney diseases (or kidney diseases that occur in days rather than weeks or months), such as blockage in the arteries to both kidneys, trauma to the kidneys, or after certain X-ray or surgical procedures. For example, certain chemicals used to observe the kidneys during an X-ray may suddenly damage the kidneys, especially in people with diabetes. Surgery that accidentally damages the arteries to the kidneys also leads to a sudden rise in blood pressure. Most of them resolve over time if the person is given the necessary medical support during the acute illness.

Testing for and treating damaged kidney tissue

Various blood and urine tests can detect damage to the kidney, but the blood tests for kidney damage don't register abnormality until a loss of more than half of the kidney tissue occurs. These tests, *blood urea nitrogen* (BUN) and *creatinine,* aren't so helpful because they only detect abnormality in the latter stages of the disease. Both of these tests measure products of normal body metabolism that should be excreted in the urine of normal kidneys. When the kidneys are damaged, these waste products back up in the blood.

On the other hand, urine can test positive for abnormal levels of protein early enough to start protecting the kidneys against further damage. An early sign of kidney tissue damage can be detected using a *microalbuminuria test,* which tests for the seeping of the protein *albumin* out of the kidney and into the urine. By looking for evidence of a tiny amount of albumin in your urine,

⤷ *Check blood test*

kidney disease can be discovered at an early stage when it's still possible to reverse it. Checking the amount of protein in the urine can be a useful test for the worsening of kidney disease because protein levels increase as more kidney tissue is lost.

A kidney *sonogram* is also useful for detecting kidney damage. A sonogram bounces sound off the kidney to evaluate its shape and size and to detect any kidney tissue loss. If the various studies don't make the diagnosis, a *biopsy* — the removal of tissue for diagnostic examination — of the kidney can often give a definitive diagnosis.

If the disease has damaged the kidneys so severely that they can no longer perform their filtering function, the kidneys are in *end-stage renal disease* (also known as kidney failure). At this point, one treatment option is *dialysis* — cleaning the blood of poisons mechanically.

While dialysis is being done, high blood pressure is present and must be controlled. Reducing the amount of fluid in the body usually accomplishes this. See Chapter 6 for more information on end-stage renal disease and dialysis.

A second treatment option is a kidney transplant. If transplantation is performed, high blood pressure can be a complication at that point as well. Transplants are less of a problem if the healthy kidney came from a person who didn't have high blood pressure. See Chapter 6 for more information on transplantation.

Certain drugs (particularly phenacetin, acetaminophen, and the nonsteroidal anti-inflammatory agents) can cause impaired kidney function. They're associated with wasting salt instead of retaining salt, so high blood pressure isn't usually a problem with these drugs.

Dealing with blocked kidney arteries

Diseases that cause *renal* (kidney) *vascular* (blood vessel) *hypertension* (high blood pressure), a block to one or both kidney arteries, bring on high blood pressure through the production of an enzyme called *renin*. The kidney that isn't receiving enough blood flow because of the obstruction secretes renin. The renin, in turn, raises the blood pressure ultimately through its action on a hormone called *angiotensin I* to produce *angiotensin II,* a hormone that causes the contraction of blood vessels. Angiotensin II also stimulates the production of *aldosterone,* a hormone that causes salt and water retention. Because of the obstruction, the increased blood pressure is still unable to cause more blood flow in the obstructed kidney, and the high blood pressure continues.

Diagnosing blocked kidney arteries

Many diseases can cause obstruction of one or both of the kidney arteries. These diseases occur in about 6 out of 100,000 people. Among them are

- ✔ **Atherosclerosis:** The process by which cholesterol is laid down in the arteries and eventually leads to narrowing of the arteries. This is usually seen in men over the age of 45 and accounts for two-thirds of cases.

- ✔ **Fibromuscular disease:** The kidney artery and the body's arteries in general becomes thickened and narrowed, especially in young women under the age of 45 and in children who have the disease.

- ✔ **Aneurysms:** The kidney artery or the heart's aorta (the artery leading to the kidney's artery) can have a defect and balloon out, thus causing blockage. Then blood enters the wall of the artery and the normal passage through which blood flows narrows. The great danger of aneurysms is bursting.

- ✔ **Emboli-clots:** Blood clots that block the artery.

A humming sound in the abdomen called a *bruit* can be a sign of these common causes of kidney artery obstruction. A bruit can be heard if the doctor listens with his stethoscope over the abdomen. This is only heard in about half of the cases, however.

Another warning sign to look for is a low potassium level in the blood. Because the kidneys produce increased amounts of the hormone aldosterone when the kidney arteries are blocked, the potassium level decreases. This diagnosis is most often associated with high blood pressure (higher than 120 diastolic) that doesn't respond to treatment.

After an artery-blocking disease is suspected, a study of the arteries to the kidneys is done. Dye is injected into the kidney arteries. The dye appears on an X-ray to show the size of the arterial passage. This can help the doctor make the diagnosis. However, if the disease has been going on for some time, even opening up the obstructed artery may not cure the high blood pressure.

Treating blocked kidney arteries

The treatment for kidney artery obstruction is artery expansion. During *angioplasty,* a type of artery expansion, a *catheter* (a slender, hollow tube) is inserted into the artery, and a balloon is used to widen it. Then a device called a *stent* is set in place to keep it open permanently.

Because renin is the cause, a drug that blocks its effect, an *angiotensin-converting enzyme* (ACE) inhibitor (see Chapter 13) can reverse the high blood pressure but may result in a fall in blood supply to the obstructed kidney. If the ACE inhibitor successfully lowers the blood pressure, then the angioplasty will most likely work. About 20 percent of the time, the disease recurs a year after the angioplasty, but results are better when the stent is used — the disease doesn't recur as often.

Hormone-Secreting Tumors That Elevate Blood Pressure

Certain tumors produce hormones (chemical messengers that trigger reactions) that elevate blood pressure to an abnormal extent. These tumors form in organs that make these hormones normally in small amounts. These tumors usually originate in an *adrenal gland,* but these tumors can also arise in nerve tissues. (You have two adrenal glands — one adrenal gland sits on top of each of your kidneys; see Figure 4-1.) The adrenal glands secrete the following hormones:

- **Epinephrine:** Maintains blood pressure and blood glucose
- **Aldosterone:** Controls salt and water levels in the bloodstream
- **Cortisol:** Maintains blood glucose (sugar) and also plays a role in maintaining blood pressure

Finding an epinephrine-producing tumor

Epinephrine (adrenaline), a normal product of the adrenal gland, raises blood pressure, heart rate, and blood glucose during stressful times and causes sweating. Sometimes a *pheochromocytoma* (a tumor that releases large quantities of epinephrine) can arise in an adrenal gland (shown with the kidneys in Figure 4-1) or along many nerves.

Figure 4-2 shows the different parts of the adrenal gland and which part is responsible for the various hormones described in this section.

Diagnosing the pheochromocytoma

Diagnosing a pheochromocytoma is rare because these epinephrine-producing tumors arise in only 6 out of 100,000 people who have high blood pressure. However, the sudden release of a large amount of epinephrine may be fatal. It's the smaller tumors that secrete the epinephrine more often. These tumors can make many other hormones and can have other symptoms depending on which hormone they're making

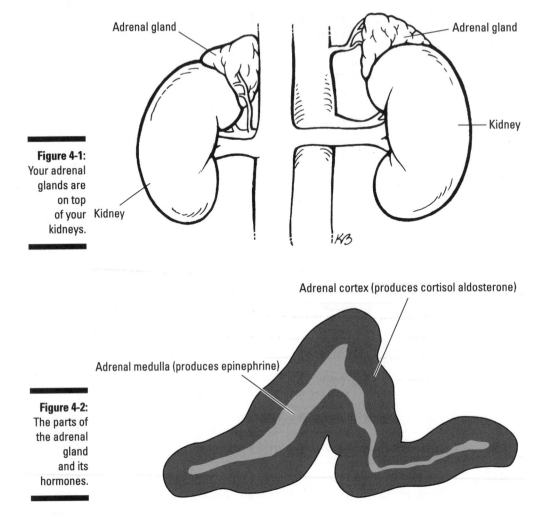

Adrenal gland

Adrenal gland

Kidney

Figure 4-1:
Your adrenal
glands are
on top
of your Kidney
kidneys.

Adrenal cortex (produces cortisol aldosterone)

Adrenal medulla (produces epinephrine)

Figure 4-2:
The parts of
the adrenal
gland
and its
hormones.

A proper diagnosis is crucial because a pheochromocytoma can cause death if the patient has some severe stress or trauma and the disease is yet undiscovered.

The key symptoms of a pheochromocytoma that are most often present are headache, *palpitations* (the feeling that the heart is beating rapidly) and excessive sweating. If high blood pressure is present, but the patient feels none of these symptoms, the diagnosis of a pheochromocytoma is extremely unlikely. High blood pressure may be intermittent, or it may be sustained in over half the patients. Exercise, urination, defecation, an enema, smoking, examination of the abdomen, and anesthesia can bring on these attacks of headache, palpitations, and sweating, which can be severe or mild at different times. The usual frequency is once a week, and the duration is less than one hour, but this can be different for each patient.

Certain cheeses, especially aged cheddar and aged Stilton, beer and wine that contain a chemical called *tyramine* may bring on a headache, palpitations, and sweating. Drugs, such as histamine, glucagons, phenothiazines, and others, can also precipitate these symptoms.

Symptoms that suggest the presence of a pheochromocytoma are present when a person is only nervous and upset and doesn't actually have a pheochromocytoma, so a pheochromocytoma is suspected much more often than it's found.

The numbered steps that follow give you an idea of what to expect if your doctor suspects an epinephrine-producing tumor.

1. **A urine test for a breakdown product of epinephrine called metanephrine is the best way to screen for a pheochromocytoma.**

   Breakdown products are the end result when the chemical is converted to an inactive form in the body.

2. **If your metanephrine level is elevated, the doctor should then ask you to collect urine for 24 hours.**

   This 24-hour urine test checks for the presence of metanephrine and *catecholamines,* which are various other breakdown products of epinephrine.

3. **After elevated levels of metanephrine and catecholamines are found, a tumor can be located with a computed tomography (CT) or magnetic resonance imaging (MRI) scan (special X-rays that are more sensitive than ordinary X-rays).**

   Most of the tumors can be found in the adrenal gland, but as noted earlier in this section, 15 percent of the time, these tumors arise in another location, such as in the nerve tissue, the abdomen, or chest cavity, which can also be seen by the scan if the tumor is large enough (more than two centimeters). The surgeon may have to find it during surgery. Usually the surgeon looks for more than the one tumor in any case. About 10 percent of the time, the tumor is malignant.

4. **If a CT or MRI scan doesn't turn up a tumor, metaiodobenzylguanidine (MIBG), a radioactive substance, is given.**

   (Try saying *metaiodobenzylguanidine* in one breath!)

   Pheochromocytomas absorb MIBG. A radiation counter is passed over the body, and when excessive radiation is found in a particular area, the tumor is localized.

Forms of pheochromocytoma run in families as solitary pheochromocytoma or along with other tumors. When several different tumors are present the condition is *multiple endocrine neoplasia* and comes in several types, each of which involves the addition of other tumors in other glands to the pheochromocytoma. Tumors of the thyroid gland and the parathyroid gland should be looked for whenever a pheochromocytoma is discovered.

Treating the pheochromocytoma

Surgery removes most pheochromocytomas, but before surgery, the patient's blood pressure has to be under control. *Dibenzyline,* a drug that blocks the action of epinephrine, may be prescribed to control the high blood pressure. A week of dibenzyline is sufficient, but if the patient has severely high blood pressure, another drug called *phentolamine* can be given in the vein every five minutes until the blood pressure is controlled and surgery can proceed.

If the blood pressure isn't controlled before surgery when a pheochromocytoma is being removed, the death rate can be as high as 50 percent. This is extremely rare, however.

The surgery is laparoscopic removal of the tumor. A small incision is made in the abdomen, a tube is inserted, and the tumor is localized and removed. (Believe me, it's not as easy as it sounds. You should watch at least a couple before trying it!) This can be done on an outpatient basis, and two weeks after surgery, the patient can return to normal activity. By comparison, the old technique of conventional surgery required five to seven days in the hospital and a four-week recovery period.

Like other secondary causes of high blood pressure, even after surgery, the high blood pressure may persist if permanent changes have occurred. Then blood pressure pills are needed.

Detecting a tumor that produces aldosterone

The *adrenal cortex* (the outer covering of the adrenal gland; see Figure 4-2) secretes *aldosterone,* an important hormone that's responsible for retaining salt and eliminating potassium from the body. A malfunction of the adrenal gland called *primary hyperaldosteronism* (usually due to an aldosterone-producing tumor in one of the adrenal glands) may produce an overabundance of aldosterone — more than the human body can handle safely. The large amount of aldosterone causes significant sodium retention and potassium loss to the point that the blood potassium is low. It also causes high blood pressure.

Similar to the prevalence of pheocromocytoma (refer to the "Diagnosing the pheochromocytoma" section, earlier in this chapter), the incidence of aldosterone-producing tumors is 2 out of 100,000 people. However, some high blood pressure specialists believe that the prevalence of primary hyperaldosteronism is much greater than generally accepted and suggest that

- ✔ As many as one in ten people with high blood pressure have primary hyperaldosteronism although not necessarily due to a tumor.
- ✔ Primary hyperaldosteronism should be considered in every case of high blood pressure even when the potassium is normal.
- ✔ Testing for the aldosterone level and the renin level in the bloodstream and getting the ratio of aldosterone to renin is recommended.

Whether this high prevalence of primary hyperaldosteronism can prove to be the case isn't clear at this time.

Diagnosing the aldosterone-producing tumor

Aldosterone-producing tumors are usually found in people between the ages of 30 and 50, and women are affected more often than men. People with an aldosterone-producing tumor have the following symptoms:

- ✔ High blood pressure (may be as high as 200/120 mm Hg)
- ✔ Increased potassium in the urine
- ✔ Increased sodium in the blood
- ✔ Increased urination (especially after lying down)
- ✔ Low potassium in the blood leading to muscle weakness

Because the blood pressure can be so high, those who suffer from an aldosterone-producing tumor may develop a brain attack, damage to the kidneys, or an enlarged heart before the disease is treated. The low potassium level in the bloodstream can lead to a reduced secretion of insulin and diabetes as well as muscle weakness.

However, sometimes a *diuretic* (see Chapter 13) is prescribed to lower the blood pressure before the aldosterone-producing tumor diagnosis is considered. Pushing potassium into the urine and thus reducing the potassium in the bloodstream are side effects of diuretics. So before an accurate conclusion can be reached concerning potassium loss, the effect of the diuretic must be removed.

Another symptom of an aldosterone-producing tumor is a low level of renin versus a significant amount of aldosterone in the bloodstream. Let me explain a little about renin to help you understand why this is so: A kidney that doesn't have sufficient blood pressure within it produces renin, an enzyme. Then as noted in the "Dealing with blocked kidney arteries" section, the renin causes production of angiotensin II from angiotensin I. Angiotensin II is a strong blood-vessel constriction agent, which also triggers the release of aldosterone. Most of the time, elevated aldosterone is secondary to increased renin. But in the case of primary hyperaldosteronism, the renin level is low while the aldosterone level is on the high side — a sign that an aldosterone-producing tumor is actually instigating the presence of aldosterone instead of renin.

The elevated blood pressure and increased blood volume result in suppression of renin production. Normally, when a person stands up, renin is released to help increase blood pressure, but in the case of this tumor, renin doesn't increase with standing.

If a person has a low blood potassium and an overabundance of potassium in the urine, a blood test for renin is done. Renin should be especially high if salt and water are withheld. If the amount of renin in your blood is, in fact, reduced, then your doctor may use that information to screen for an aldosterone-producing tumor. If the level of renin is low, the aldosterone level is measured, preferably in the early morning because aldosterone tends to fall at night, even from a tumor. If the aldosterone level is high, the diagnosis is an aldosterone-secreting tumor or *bilateral adrenal hyperplasia* — increased aldosterone production in both adrenals as a result of having many nodules. This is an important distinction because bilateral adrenal hyperplasia tends to be a milder disease than a tumor, and it doesn't respond well to surgery.

After the chemical studies show that aldosterone is being made to excess in the presence of low renin, a CT or MRI scan is done to separate a solitary adrenal tumor from bilateral hyperplasia. Occasionally, this study doesn't make the distinction. This is because aldosterone-producing tumors tend to be small and the incidence of innocent growths called *incidentalomas* on the adrenal gland is high. Then the radiologist puts a tube into the adrenal veins on each side of the body and looks for the side that has large amounts of aldosterone in the sample.

Treating the aldosterone-producing tumor

The treatment of a solitary adrenal tumor that makes too much aldosterone is surgery using the technique of laparoscopy. The affected individual isn't opened with a large incision but has tubes placed into the abdomen. The tumor is found and removed through the tube. Before surgery to remove the tumor is performed, *spironolactone,* a drug that reverses the action of aldosterone, is prescribed to make the patient normal chemically. After the surgery is done, the aldosterone level falls, the potassium returns to normal, and the blood pressure returns to normal as well. Sometimes the blood pressure stays up because the patient also has *essential high blood pressure* (high blood pressure for which the cause can't be determined) or because permanent damage has taken place in the blood vessels or the kidneys. This is true most often for individuals who've had high blood pressure for five years or longer.

Lapping up licorice can lower your renin

Believe it or not — eating lots of licorice can raise your blood pressure and lower the amount of renin in your bloodstream. People who eat an abundance of licorice block the action of an enzyme in the kidney that converts cortisol to cortisone. While cortisol has some activity similar to aldosterone, cortisone doesn't. The unusually high concentrations of cortisol in the kidney cause a clinical picture that imitates aldosterone excess. However, the history of licorice eating can be obtained and the aldosterone is low — not high in this case. Don't worry though: It usually takes four weeks of eating large quantities (50 to 100 grams) of licorice to produce this condition.

Medical treatment of a single tumor with a drug that reverses the action of aldosterone isn't usually done, particularly in men, because the treatment drug of choice, spironolactone, has significant side effects including breast enlargement, reduced interest in sex, and reduced ability to have an erection. Many patients with a single tumor, however, can't undergo surgery or refuse surgery. In this situation, medical treatment has been successful for five years or more.

Bilateral adrenal hyperplasia, where both adrenal glands are large and making too much aldosterone, is treated medically with spironolactone. This is because removal of the adrenal glands doesn't generally cure the high blood pressure even though the low potassium improves.

Managing Cushing's Syndrome

As if the previous two tumors weren't enough trouble from the adrenal gland, the adrenal gland can be the site of still another source of secondary high blood pressure, namely *Cushing's syndrome.* This syndrome results whenever the adrenal glands make too much cortisol. This can occur in three different ways:

- ✔ The pituitary hormone that regulates the adrenal gland stimulates the adrenals.
- ✔ A tumor grows within one adrenal gland.
- ✔ Rarely, an adrenal-stimulating hormone coming from some other tumor in the body stimulates the adrenals.

The overabundance of cortisol usually (about 80 percent of the time) results from an excessive production of *adrenocorticotrophin* (ACTH) — the hormone that regulates the adrenal glands — coming from the pituitary gland in the brain. The ACTH stimulates both adrenals to make too much cortisol.

The remaining 20 percent of the time, one adrenal gland has a tumor within it that makes too much cortisol (the main hormone made by the adrenal glands). Normally, the adrenal gland is under the control of ACTH from the brain. If a tumor forms in the part of the brain that makes ACTH, the pituitary gland, it can cause the adrenals to make too much cortisol as well as other steroids that have plenty of salt-retaining activity, and thus the blood pressure rises. When the adrenal tumor makes too much cortisol independently of ACTH, ACTH is suppressed instead of elevated.

Diagnosing the presence of Cushing's syndrome

Cushing's syndrome is associated with high blood pressure that's difficult to treat. The pressure may be up to 200/120 mm Hg. The death rate from untreated Cushing's syndrome is high. It occurs three times as often in women as men, usually in the third or fourth decade of an individual's life.

Too much cortisol in the bloodstream has other properties that may result in

✔ Diabetes mellitus

✔ Easy bruising of the body

✔ Loss of bone with spontaneous fractures

✔ Obesity of the trunk of the body with thin arms and legs

✔ Psychological changes ranging from irritability to severe depression

✔ Stretch marks, especially on the abdomen

In addition, the high ACTH and the pituitary tumor that it represents can cause still other symptoms. Some of these signs and symptoms besides high blood pressure are

✔ Headache caused by the pituitary tumor

✔ Pigmentation of the body and any stretch marks caused by the ACTH

✔ Loss of menstrual function in women caused by other hormones made by the adrenals in excess that have masculinizing properties

✔ Hairiness in women caused by the same masculinizing hormones

With all these signs and symptoms in addition to the high blood pressure, the diagnosis of Cushing's syndrome is often considered. After the diagnosis is made, it's relatively easy to prove it with chemical tests.

The best screening test for Cushing's syndrome is one milligram of *dexamethasone,* a steroid hormone much like cortisol, taken at midnight. If Cushing's syndrome is not present, that one milligram is enough to shut down ACTH such that the amount of cortisol in the bloodstream is low when tested the following morning. However, when a pituitary tumor makes ACTH or an independent tumor of the adrenal gland makes cortisol, the dexamethasone can't shut down cortisol production, and the next morning, cortisol is still elevated.

Another confirmatory study is a 24-hour urine collection for cortisol, which should be high when Cushing's syndrome is present.

If the screening test with dexamethasone is positive, a test using a higher dose of dexamethasone for a longer time can absolutely confirm the diagnosis. Then another test that measures the amount of ACTH in the bloodstream is administered. If these test results show that the level of ACTH is high, then a pituitary tumor is suspected. But if test results reveal that the level of ACTH is low, then an adrenal tumor is most likely the case.

Sometimes ACTH can come from another source than the pituitary, usually some other type of tumor, particularly a lung cancer. This is *ectopic* (from an abnormal site) ACTH production. The result is Cushing's syndrome again, but it tends to be more aggressive, and the ectopic source often has some symptom that points to it. The use of dexamethasone in a still higher dose separates pituitary ACTH overproduction (which is finally suppressed with enough dexamethasone) from ectopic ACTH overproduction, which is not suppressed at all.

After the source of the excess cortisol is determined, a CT or MRI is done on the pituitary if ACTH is high or the adrenals if ACTH is low. If an ectopic source of ACTH is suspected, the CT is directed to look for a tumor in the chest and the abdomen.

Treating Cushing's syndrome

The first step in treating Cushing's syndrome is to control the blood pressure with drugs. After this is accomplished, the treatment is directed to the source of the excess hormone. If the pituitary is responsible through an ACTH-producing tumor, an operation is performed under anesthesia (don't worry, you won't feel a thing) that involves passing a tube through the nose into the pituitary gland for the removal of the tumor. If this isn't successful or feasible, X-ray therapy to the pituitary is done.

Sometimes the pituitary can't be treated if, for example, the patient refuses surgery. Then both adrenal glands are removed because the hormones from the adrenals are responsible for most of the signs and symptoms. After this is done, the patient is treated with steroid replacement. A complication of this form of treatment is the increasing growth of the tumor in the pituitary making an abundance of ACTH, resulting in significant darkening of the skin that takes ten years or more to develop after the removal of both adrenals — a condition known as *Nelson's syndrome*. Then the pituitary tumor must be removed.

If the adrenal gland has a tumor that makes too much cortisol independent of ACTH control, that tumor is removed in much the same way that an aldosterone-producing tumor is removed. (See the "Treating the aldosterone-producing tumor" section, earlier in this chapter.)

If ACTH has an ectopic source, then the ACTH is often from a cancer, and chemotherapy may be necessary.

After a tumor is removed, the patient may have a period as long as six months when the cortisol is abnormally low and has to be supported by taking replacement medication. At that point, the cortisol can be phased out and the patient's own adrenal gland takes over. Table 4-1 sums up the treatment for these various forms of Cushing's syndrome.

Table 4-1	Forms of Cushing's Syndrome and Their Treatment
Site of Tumor	*Treatment Used*
Pituitary gland	Remove pituitary tumor
Adrenal gland	Remove adrenal tumor
Ectopic source of ACTH	Locate and remove ectopic source

Realizing a Genetic Disease is Causing High Blood Pressure

Congenital adrenal hyperplasia, an inherited disease, is the genetic lack of one or more enzymes that are needed to change steroids from one form to another and eventually to cortisol in the adrenal glands. This leads to an overproduction of other hormones that have properties similar to aldosterone. When the pituitary gland does not detect sufficient cortisol, it sends out more ACTH to stimulate the adrenals, which then enlarge. The two most common forms of congenital adrenal hyperplasia are discussed as follows.

✔ In one form of congenital adrenal hyperplasia, the excessive steroids are both aldosterone-like, producing high blood pressure and low potassium, and masculinizing, causing masculine changes in baby girls, so that their genital organs are something between male and female. A milder form can present itself in such a way that the onset of puberty in boys is early. The symptomatic increase of male hormone activity, such as increased hair and menstrual irregularity, can also occur in young girls.

✔ In a second form of congenital adrenal hyperplasia, the excessive steroids are again aldosterone-like, causing high blood pressure and low potassium, but no sex hormones are made at all. When the female is supposed to begin menstruation, it doesn't take place, so the disease is first detected at puberty. Lack of male hormone in boys leads to abnormal development of the male sexual organs, which is found earlier than in the case of the girls.

Although these conditions are rare, they're easily treated if diagnosed early. The patients are simply given cortisol, which shuts off the excessive ACTH and the production of the abnormal steroids. In the second form of congenital adrenal hyperplasia, sex hormones must be given to replace the absent hormones. Because these diseases are hereditary, they're found in certain groups more often than others. This alerts doctors to look for the condition whenever a new birth occurs in one of these groups.

Other Causes of Secondary High Blood Pressure

Several other treatable diseases can be associated with high blood pressure. These diseases need to be considered because most of them are reversible, and the high blood pressure responds to the correction of the disease unless it's been present for some time.

Coarctation of the aorta

Coarctation of the aorta is a narrowing of the large artery that leaves the heart. Depending on how severe the narrowing is, the narrowing is usually present at birth though not diagnosed until the teenage years. The narrowing is usually in an area soon after the beginning of the aorta but below where the artery branches off to supply blood to the arms. The result is that the blood pressure in the arms is high and the blood pressure in the legs is lower.

The kidneys are also exposed to the lower blood pressure and respond by putting out more of the enzyme renin, leading to even higher blood pressure above the narrowing but not below it.

The narrowing results in the production of a sound called a *murmur,* a humming sound, which can be heard with the doctor's stethoscope in the area of the heart. Measuring the blood pressure in the arms followed by measuring it in the legs shows the difference. When the pulse is looked for in the groin, where it is usually felt, no pulse can be detected.

Children with this condition can have nosebleeds, dizziness, pounding headaches, and leg cramps with exercise.

During a careful first examination of the baby, the doctor feels for the pulses in the feet and notes if the pulses are present or not. If not felt, further evaluation is done with a CT or MRI of the chest.

The treatment consists of opening the narrow area with surgery, or sometimes the same technique is used for opening the blood vessels of the heart when they're narrowed — a procedure known as *balloon angioplasty.* (See the "Treating blocked kidney arteries" section, earlier in this chapter for more on angioplasty.) If it's not treated, the patient may die before the age of 40 from complications of high blood pressure.

Too much or too little thyroid hormone

Both *hyperthyroidism* (too much thyroid hormone) and *hypothyroidism* (too little thyroid hormone) can be associated with high blood pressure. These conditions may be easy to diagnose if the symptoms are significant, but hypothyroidism is often subtle.

If the patient has high cholesterol in addition to high blood pressure, the diagnosis of hypothyroidism should certainly be considered.

If the patient has a rapid pulse, weight loss, and sweating in addition to the high blood pressure, then hyperthyroidism must be considered.

Screening for thyroid disease is simple. Thyroid disease is so common that everyone over age 35 should have a screening blood test. For more information on your thyroid, see my book *Thyroid For Dummies* (Wiley). Screening consists of a thyroid-stimulating hormone level blood test. If the hormone level is low, then hyperthyroidism may be present. If the hormone level is high, then hypothyroidism is the diagnosis.

Ask your doctor to screen you for thyroid disease beginning at age 35 and every five years thereafter.

Hyperthyroidism and hypothyroidism can be treated easily after the diagnosis is made. Pills to block thyroid hormone production or a dose of radioactive iodine can control hyperthyroidism. Replacement thyroid hormone by mouth can cure hypothyroidism. (Replacement thyroid hormone cures hypothyroidism so that the person is entirely normal with the exception of the need for a pill daily. That's as good a cure as I know.) The blood pressure returns to normal after either disease is treated.

Acromegaly

Acromegaly results from a slow-growing tumor of the pituitary gland that makes too much growth hormone. Among other things, the growth hormone causes sodium retention and high blood pressure.

Acromegaly causes many other signs besides high blood pressure. The patient has a characteristic appearance. If the disease begins before the bones close (a person grows taller until the growing ends of bones are eliminated, referred to as the *bones closing*), the patient is extremely tall, often unable to get through doors without stooping way down. The hands and the feet grow thick. The skin is coarse and oily. The lips, nose, and tongue are thick as well. Acromegaly patients are weak and sweat excessively. The conditions that result in early death due to acromegaly if it's untreated are diabetes, high blood pressure, and heart disease.

Acromegaly is diagnosed by testing the blood for growth hormone at a time when it should be low after taking in glucose, the type of sugar in the blood. If elevated growth hormone is found, the next step is a CT of the brain to look for a pituitary tumor. Sometimes, other tumors in the body produce growth hormone, and the pituitary appears normal.

Drugs are available to treat acromegaly, but they're not entirely successful and are associated with side effects. Instead, after a pituitary tumor is found, surgery is usually recommended. A brain surgeon goes in through the nose and removes the tumor. If the surgery is successful, the skin shows improvement in a few days. It's most successful when the level of growth hormone isn't high.

When surgery is ineffective, radiation to the pituitary is often done and can cure the disease, but it may also cause loss of other pituitary functions, such as the production of the hormones that control the thyroid gland, the adrenal gland, and the genital organs. The blood pressure does fall when the level of growth hormone is made normal.

Sleep apnea

Sleep apnea is a condition in which an individual gasps for breath and snores during sleep following several stops in breathing. It's significant when it happens five or more times in an hour. The result of the extremely restless sleep is that the person is extremely tired during the day, has headaches, and tends to fall asleep at times when he doesn't want to, such as driving a car and during work.

Because the lack of breathing occurs many times, the person has a reduction in blood oxygen and an increase in carbon dioxide in the blood. The decrease in oxygen causes constriction of the blood vessels with resultant high blood pressure. These people have also been found to have increased heart disease.

Sleep apnea is diagnosed in a sleep laboratory where doctors can observe the person sleeping, snoring, and failing to breathe for many periods of time. After the diagnosis is made, the person can be given a machine attached to a mask that's worn over the face and provides positive pressure. This keeps the airway open so that periods of breathing loss don't occur, and the loud snoring doesn't occur because the individual doesn't have to gasp for breath. Sleeping is much more restful, and the person doesn't fall asleep during the day. The high blood pressure usually subsides as well.

If the condition has gone on for a long time, the high blood pressure may continue, and pills may be required to control it.

Brain tumor

Brain tumors increase pressure within the brain and the blood pressure throughout the body. The blood pressure rise may not be constant and may mimic a pheochromocytoma. (See more on pheochromocytomas in the "Finding an epinephrine-producing tumor" section, earlier in this chapter.) If the brain tumor can be managed successfully, the high blood pressure returns to normal. If not, blood pressure pills are required to control it.

Burns

Severe burns are associated with high blood pressure in about 25 percent of burn cases. The high stress associated with the burn causes the high blood pressure. A bad burn also triggers the release of hormones that cause blood vessel constriction. If the patient survives the burn, the blood pressure returns to normal after about two weeks.

Part II
Considering the Medical Consequences

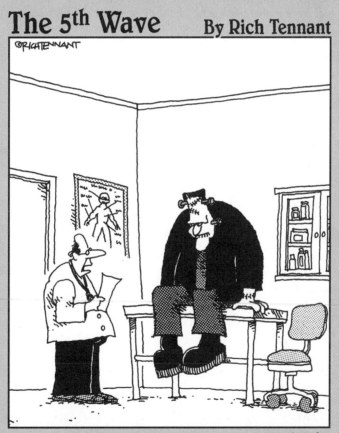

The 5th Wave   By Rich Tennant

"It's important that you get your high blood pressure under control. It could not only affect your kidneys and heart, but also your current brain."

In this part . . .

Three major organs of the body suffer when high blood pressure isn't controlled: the heart, the kidneys, and the brain. In this part, I explain exactly how high blood pressure affects each of these organs and how the sooner any damage is diagnosed, the better the chances are of reversing the damage. I also address ways to deal with organ damage that may have already resulted from high blood pressure.

Although I separate these three major organs into three separate chapters in this part, unfortunately, uncontrolled high blood pressure doesn't pick and choose. Uncontrolled high blood pressure tends to damage all these organs together and within the same time frame.

Chapter 5

Pumping Your Blood: The Heart

• •

In This Chapter

▶ Following your blood through the heart

▶ Looking at various diseases that affect the heart

▶ Figuring out when your heart is failing and how

▶ Eliminating bad habits

• •

*H*eart disease is the leading cause of death throughout the world. Heart disease involves the muscles of the heart and the blood vessels that provide nutrition to those muscles. Various forms of heart disease include chest pain caused by a decreased blood supply to the heart (called *angina*), heart attacks, and heart failure. High blood pressure plays a major role in the development of heart disease.

High blood pressure is rarely found without other risk factors, such as diabetes, smoking, and lack of exercise. These risk factors, when mixed in with high blood pressure, can increase the chance of a fatal heart attack as much as 15 to 20 times. People with untreated high blood pressure may live 10 to 20 years less than people without high blood pressure. If the blood pressure is controlled consistently, a person's life span isn't shortened.

It's been said that gambling is a great way of getting nothing for something, and you can gamble away your life if you don't control your blood pressure — this is guaranteed. You must make up your mind to get something for something. Take the trouble to measure your blood pressure properly and to follow the recommendations in Part III, and I guarantee that you'll not only live longer, but you'll increase the quality of your life — free of much of the medical misery that people develop as they get older.

This chapter tells you what you need to know about high blood pressure and your heart. It provides a foundation for moving into Part III. If you read this whole chapter, you'll have an excellent understanding of the importance of blood pressure control especially for your heart. The other chapters in this part also provide an understanding how high blood pressure affects your kidneys and your brain.

The heart, kidneys, and brain are discussed in three separate chapters, but uncontrolled high blood pressure triggers the development of heart disease, kidney disease, and a brain attack all at the same time.

Introducing the Mighty Pump

What a piece of work is the heart! An organ that's mostly muscle, your heart is about the size of your clenched fist and weighs about 10½ ounces. This little muscle is responsible for supplying blood and oxygen to all parts of your body, which is usually 15 or more times as heavy as the heart itself.

Your heart is in your chest cavity behind your breastbone and between your lungs. The heart is divided into four chambers, the left and right atria and the left and right ventricles. The right atrium receives blood through the veins called *vena cava* and pushes it into the right ventricle. The right ventricle squeezes down and sends the blood into the pulmonary arteries to the lungs where the blood picks up oxygen. Pulmonary veins carry the blood back to the left atrium, which sends it down to the left ventricle. The left ventricle squeezes the blood into a major artery, the aorta, which sends it to every cell and organ. Valves that close, blocking backward flow, prevent the blood from going backwards from the left side of the heart to the lungs, from the right side of the heart to the veins, and from the ventricles to the atria.

This amazing pump pushes 1½ gallons of blood forward every minute. Every hour, it sends 90 gallons around the body, enough to fill the gas tanks in most cars six times, assuming a 15-gallon gas tank. In a day that you spend mostly resting, your heart pumps 2,160 gallons of blood. If you're working or playing energetically, the number gets much higher.

The combination of the heart, the blood vessels that carry the blood, and the blood itself is the *cardiovascular system.*

When the blood pressure rises, the heart must work harder to push the blood through. It was not meant to have to struggle so hard and eventually it may fail, a condition where the heart muscles are just too tired and weak to work properly.

Blocking Blood Flow to the Heart Muscle

Just like any other organ of the body, your heart muscle must receive oxygen, *glucose* (blood sugar), and other nutrients in order to work. These nutrients are the food of the heart muscles. When the bloodstream that carries these nutrients is partially obstructed (called *arteriosclerosis*) so that the heart muscle is partially starving, the heart muscle can cause pain. (For more on arteriosclerosis, see the "Examining arteriosclerosis" section coming up next in this chapter.) If the obstruction remains about the same, the pain is stable. A complete obstruction causes a heart attack, which is the death of heart muscle tissue.

Examining arteriosclerosis

Arteriosclerosis is hardening of the arteries — the process that leads to obstruction of arteries throughout the body as a result of deposition of cholesterol and formation of a plaque, a narrowing of an artery that blocks the flow of blood. (See the "Formation of a plaque" sidebar in this chapter.) When the blood flow is blocked, the heart has to pump harder, leading to thickening of the heart muscles called *hypertrophy*.

High blood pressure can increase the development of fatty deposits in the walls of the arteries leading to

- **Atherosclerosis:** A form of arteriosclerosis in the medium- to large-size arteries
- **Arteriolosclerosis:** Arteriosclerosis in the small arteries
- **Coronary atherosclerosis:** Involves the arteries to the muscle of the heart

As the coronary arteries (the ones that feed the heart muscle) become more and more blocked, the heart muscle may be hungry for nutrients or even die, a condition called *coronary artery disease* (also known as *coronary heart disease* and *atherosclerotic heart disease*).

According to the National Institutes of Health, one of every five deaths (460,000 total) in the United States each year is the result of atherosclerosis of the arteries to the heart, resulting in a lethal heart attack. In addition to these deaths, another 650,000 people have heart attacks but don't die for a total of about 1.1 million. About 12½ million people in the United States have chest pain associated with coronary atherosclerosis, a heart attack, or some other form of coronary atherosclerosis. Due to the greater prevalence of high blood pressure among the African American population, this group has a higher rate of coronary heart disease than any other ethnic group.

Formation of a plaque

When high blood pressure, smoking, diabetes and/or increased levels of cholesterol, especially low-density lipoprotein (LDL) cholesterol, damage the inner lining of the arteries, a plaque begins to form. The following figure shows the parts of a normal artery and the artery after a plaque has developed.

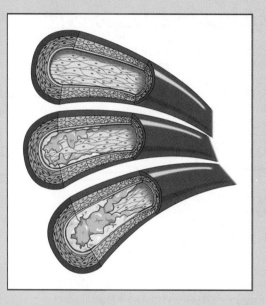

After damage has occurred, fat begins to accumulate within a part of the artery wall called the *intima.* In the intima, fat is protected from the chemicals in the blood that prevent changes in the fat, and it begins to change to a more damaging form.

White blood cells, especially monocytes and lymphocytes that enter the intima from the blood, are transformed into other cells called *macrophages,* and the macrophages begin gobbling up the changed fat to turn the cells into *foam cells.* Calcium is also deposited in the walls where the plaque is forming and is responsible for the calcification seen in arteries when X-rays are taken.

This accumulation of foam cells and calcium is now called plaque. It grows and begins to stick out into the *lumen* (the hollow part inside) of the artery. After 80 percent of the lumen is blocked, blood flow to the heart muscle is reduced.

The irregular surface of a plaque can be the site of accumulation of blood platelets and the formation of a clot. The clot can go on and reduce the opening of the lumen even more at that position, or it can break off and lodge in a smaller artery, completely closing off blood flow beyond it.

Atherosclerotic heart disease (coronary artery disease) is found in the arteries of people who die as young as age twenty, or even younger of other causes, and is extensive in older people who die of other causes. However, it's not found in everyone. Those who don't have risk factors, such as uncontrolled high blood pressure, cigarette smoking, diabetes, a sedentary lifestyle, and high cholesterol levels, rarely have problems with coronary artery disease. A family history of coronary artery disease is another risk factor and one that you can do nothing about, but its effect is minimized when the other risk factors are avoided or controlled.

Coronary artery disease may cause sudden death as the first sign of the presence of the disease in as many as 25 percent of the patients. Another 20 percent die before they reach the hospital as a result of a fatal irregularity in their heartbeat. The rest may undergo a procedure to try to open the blocked artery or arteries. (See the "Opting for surgery" section coming up later in this chapter.)

A large group of patients with coronary artery disease have a relatively stable form of chest pain discussed in the next section, "Managing stable heart pain."

Managing stable heart pain

Stable heart pain, pain that doesn't get worse over time, due to coronary atherosclerosis, is *angina pectoris* (Latin for "pain in the chest"). Angina pectoris (commonly known as *angina*) affects 6.5 million people in the United States. Not only is angina pectoris the result of blockage of an artery, but it can also be brought on if the coronary artery squeezes down, for example, after a meal when blood is diverted to the intestine, thus causing a decrease in blood supply to the heart. Some diseases like hyperthyroidism (stemming from an overactive thyroid gland), which increases the demands on the body's metabolism, can cause angina even in the absence of coronary atherosclerosis. Figure 5-1 shows the location of the major arteries that provide blood supply to the heart muscles. The right coronary artery supplies blood to the right side of the heart. The left main coronary artery supplies the left side of the heart. It, in turn, divides into the left anterior descending artery that supplies the front of the left side and the left circumflex artery that curves around to the back. Both the left and right coronary arteries begin as the left ventricle continues into the aorta, the major artery carrying blood away from the heart to the rest of the body.

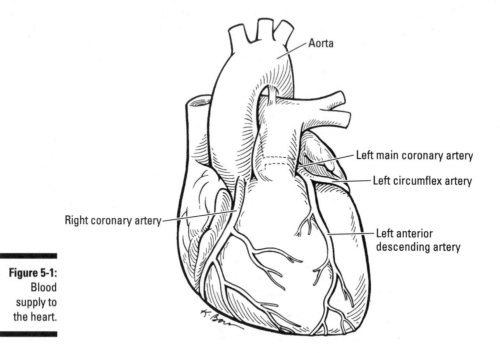

Aorta

Left main coronary artery

Left circumflex artery

Right coronary artery

Left anterior descending artery

Figure 5-1:
Blood
supply to
the heart.

Identifying the symptoms and making a diagnosis

Some of the characteristic symptoms of coronary artery disease include the following:

- ✔ Chest pain begins with activity and is relieved with rest. The pain is most often felt in the front of the chest on the left side and radiates down the left arm. After a meal or during excitement, it takes less activity to bring on the pain. Strong emotions can bring on pain even without activity.

- ✔ Symptomatic "pain" in the chest may be absent. However, according to coronary artery disease patients, symptomatic discomfort in the chest area can include burning, squeezing, pressing, aching, or indigestion.

- ✔ The area of discomfort is most often behind the middle of the chest and tends to be felt in the same area in each individual. Some of the other places it may be felt include the right side of the chest, the left shoulder, and sometimes the right shoulder. It can also be felt in the jaw. It often radiates from one of those sites back to the chest.

- ✔ Discomfort may last no longer than a few minutes, especially if the patient rests as soon as it starts. It doesn't last longer than 30 minutes.

- ✔ Nitroglycerin often brings about a response in the form of pain reduction or cessation. This response helps to make the diagnosis.

The patient's description of symptoms usually leads the doctor to diagnose angina. The classic way to make a diagnosis of angina pectoris is with a stress test. The patient walks on a treadmill or bikes on a stable bike rapidly for up to 12 minutes at increasing speeds and increasing slopes of the treadmill while a continuous *electrocardiogram* (EKG), a recording of the electrical impulses in the heart, is performed. It's accurate only if the patient achieves a certain level of activity and heart rate and sustains the activity long enough. Especially if chest pain occurs during the EKG, the doctor looks for specific changes on the graph paper.

After a stress test indicates that angina pectoris is present, other tests that don't require invading the patient's body more than an intravenous line are performed to further characterize the severity of the coronary artery disease including

- **Myocardial perfusion scan:** This shows where the heart muscle, the myocardium, is receiving normal blood flow and where this is reduced due to reduced blood flow. A radioactive tracer is injected through an IV and an instrument like a Geiger counter for detecting radioactivity finds where the tracer localizes in the heart.

- **Radionuclide angiography:** Measures the ejection fraction (or the ratio of the amount of blood that's pushed out of the heart with each beat) and the motion of the heart wall, indicating which areas may have lost their blood supply and are probably dead tissue. The ejection fraction should rise with exercise, but when coronary artery disease is present, it may fall. A radioactive substance is injected into your blood through an IV that attaches to red blood cells. The radioactivity is counted as it goes through your heart.

- **Echocardiography:** Using sound to bounce off the walls of the heart, this test shows areas that don't contract along with the rest of the heart muscle. A device is held over your heart that sends a sound wave to the heart muscle producing a picture of the moving heart muscle. This is truly "noninvasive" to your body.

- **Coronary angiogram:** This is the gold standard for the diagnosis of angina pectoris, and it's done when the preceding tests indicate an abnormality. This involves placing a catheter in the individual coronary arteries and injecting a dye that can be seen on X-ray to find the areas of narrowing. Coronary angiography isn't done on all patients with angina but only for patients who exhibit the following:

  - Stable angina (chest pain that doesn't get worse over time) or unstable angina (chest pain that worsens over time) is present, and medical treatment with pills is unsuccessful.

  - Symptoms don't point to a diagnosis of coronary artery disease.

- Coronary artery surgery has been performed, but symptoms return.

- Heart has severe abnormal rhythm disturbances that may be caused by coronary artery disease.

After a coronary angiogram clearly points to obstructive coronary artery disease as the cause of the symptoms, the decision must be made as to the type of treatment.

Treating with medication

Three major forms of treatment are available for coronary artery obstruction, and each has its advantages and disadvantages. One treatment option for patients with stable, uncomplicated angina pectoris is medication. This option is usually best for patients who aren't interested in exertion. However, if the patient is interested in being able to perform energetic activities or has unstable angina, then PTCA or CABG is the treatment of choice. (PTCA and CABG involve surgery and are discussed in the "Opting for surgery" section later in this chapter.)

Before drugs are prescribed, the first step is to eliminate contributing factors. (See "Avoiding the Risk Factors" later in this chapter.) If blood pressure is high, it must be brought under control. It the patient is smoking, he must stop. Diabetes should be controlled, and an elevated cholesterol should be treated. Strenuous activity may provoke pain, and this may have to be eliminated as well.

A number of drugs have successfully reduced pain and increased the time that such patients can exercise without pain. For example:

- **Nitroglycerin** has been successful for years. It opens up the arteries directly and also lowers the blood pressure, so that the heart doesn't have to work as hard. Nitroglycerin is taken under the tongue at the first sign of pain and usually works in minutes.

- **Long-acting nitrates,** such as isosorbide dinitrate and isosorbide mononitrate, decrease the frequency of pain attacks. They can also be administered in a patch that's worn during the day so that the drug is absorbed through the skin.

- **Beta blockers,** a class of drugs that include propranolol, metoprolol, and atenolol, decrease the heart's oxygen requirements, thereby decreasing pain. Beta blockers actually prolong the life of angina sufferers.

- **Calcium channel blocking agents,** another class of drugs, such as verapamil and diltiazem, also reduce the heart's oxygen needs by reducing blood pressure and heart rate.

- **Drugs that dilate the blood vessels and drugs,** such as aspirin, that prevent the blood's platelets from joining together to form a clot can reduce pain and prevent further clotting.

Opting for surgery

Two surgical procedures that treat coronary artery obstruction include *percutaneous transluminal coronary angioplasty,* conveniently shortened to PTCA, and *coronary artery bypass graft* (CABG).

Studies of patients who were randomly given PTCA or CABG show that the results are similar. For a single blocked blood vessel, there is no difference in the rate of success of the operation. This is true for multiple vessels as well, so long as the patients aren't diabetic and the obstructed blood vessels can be entered. In the latter cases, bypass surgery is the treatment of choice.

During the PTCA procedure, a flexible wire is passed through the *lumen* (the hollow part inside) of the artery past the area of obstruction. A balloon is passed along the wire and into the obstruction where it's repeatedly inflated and deflated until the obstruction is significantly reduced. Because of the high rate of recurrence of the obstruction in the past, a small flexible stent, made of stainless steel and often covered with polyester is currently inserted at the point of obstruction to keep it open.

A CABG involves cutting and reattaching one or both of the arteries to the breasts (the internal mammary arteries) to deliver blood to the coronary artery past the point of an obstruction. Another CABG technique takes a vein from the leg and grafts it onto the aorta, the large blood vessel coming out of the heart, and to a point past the obstruction of a coronary artery. As many as five bypasses are performed at one surgery.

PTCA has a number of advantages as compared to CAGB:

- ✔ For an experienced surgeon, PTCA is an simpler surgery, and it doesn't require anesthesia.

- ✔ The chest isn't opened up.

- ✔ The heart isn't bypassed as surgery is done.

- ✔ Convalescence is relatively short, and the usual discharge occurs after 24 hours.

CAGB — which requires anesthesia, opening of the chest, bypassing the heart, and a prolonged convalescence — is a more involved procedure than PTCA. However, in general, the treatment lasts longer and provides a more complete reopening of blood flow. Recent advances in CABG that have eliminated the need to bypass the heart and the lungs have made the procedure even more appealing.

Disadvantages and complications accompany each procedure. For example, PTCA can't be performed when an artery is completely closed. Also, if many separate lesions are present, PTCA isn't effective. This may be the reason that PTCA isn't considered the treatment of choice for coronary artery disease in diabetes. These patients do much better with CABG.

CABG can also have complications, such as an acute heart attack, a stroke, an infection in the area of the body that surgery is being performed on, and even death on the operating table, especially in older patients (more than 70 years old), and those patients with other diseases, such as kidney disease and diabetes. In these patients, CABG is only done on the most symptomatic.

Treating an acute heart attack

A heart attack, also known as a *myocardial infarction* (MI), where heart muscle tissue dies because it lacks a supply of blood, can cause immediate death in 25 percent of the people who have one, and another 20 percent never reach the hospital alive. For those who do make it to the hospital, however, excellent treatment is available.

The symptoms that suggest that an individual is having a heart attack include the following:

- Development of severe pain in the front of the chest that lasts for more than 30 minutes with radiation down the left arm
- Unexplained shock, a severe fall in blood pressure, sometimes accompanied by vomiting and even unconsciousness
- A feeling of impending doom with sweating and a rapid heart beat

Call 911 for an ambulance ride to the nearest hospital, and call your doctor for follow-up.

The doctor will question you to find out if there has been a recent change in your pattern of chest pain. He'll ask whether you're experiencing sweating, dizziness, nausea, and weakness.

Your blood pressure may be low. You may appear pale. Your heart rhythm may be irregular. On examination, your chest may have *rales,* the sound of fluid in the lungs as a result of some *heart failure* (when your heart isn't able to pump enough blood to maintain an adequate flow to and from the body tissues). Your heart may reveal soft sounds that mean the muscle isn't functioning properly.

The doctor does lab studies, which may show the following:

- Elevations of heart enzymes, chemicals usually found only in the heart that leak into the blood when the heart muscle is damaged.
- Electrocardiographic changes that suggest a heart attack
- Changes in the movement of the heart wall, so that when the wall should be moving in to squeeze out blood, it doesn't move or flops outward.

One of the biggest advances in the treatment of heart attacks is the availability of *thrombolytic therapy,* drugs that dissolve the clot that's obstructing the coronary artery and that allow blood to flow back into the obstructed area. This decreases the size of the damage and often saves the patient. A possible side effect of thrombolytic therapy is the danger of bleeding in undesired areas such as the brain, especially if the blood pressure isn't controlled.

Several different agents are used for thrombolytic therapy. The choice depends on your doctor's experience with each of them. The success of this treatment depends on how quickly the patient gets to the doctor after the onset of the heart attack, and the earlier, the better. The reopening may be as much as 80 percent. This reopening accompanies an end to the pain and an improved EKG reading.

The blood vessel closes again in 10 percent of cases, and then PTCA or CABG surgery must be done to permanently reopen the artery. (PTCA and CABG are described earlier in this chapter in the "Opting for surgery" section.) Sometimes the thrombolytic therapy isn't done in favor of immediate PTCA, especially in the severely sick patient with a heart attack and shock.

After the initial treatment is given, the heart attack patient is observed in the coronary care unit for a couple of days. Then the patient gradually returns to normal activity. Studies have shown that several drugs can significantly reduce the chance of a future heart attack when they're prescribed early. Aspirin is administered to prevent more clots. Beta blockers have been shown to extend the life of the patient after a heart attack. If pain occurs, nitroglycerine remains the treatment of choice.

Developing Heart Failure

When high blood pressure is present, your heart is forced to pump against more resistance. It needs to sustain its output, so it must thicken to do so. Just like the muscles of a weight lifter, the heart muscle gets bigger and thicker. But heart muscle can only thicken so far. After a while, the heart enlarges to the point that it can no longer pump effectively and heart failure begins.

Comparing the statistics for the prevalence of heart failure today with 20 years ago, clearly, more heart failure is occurring today. Exactly why this is so isn't clear, but uncontrolled high blood pressure is certainly one contributing factor.

If you suffer from heart failure, you may experience angina pectoris (pain most often felt in the front of the chest) or it can be felt in the jaw, the left arm, or the shoulder. (Angina is described earlier in this chapter in the "Managing stable heart pain" section.) This comes from the high oxygen requirement of the thick heart muscle plus the decreased blood supply coming through the arteries that supply the heart. At first, angina pain begins during activity. As the condition worsens, it occurs when you're at rest.

Your doctor can tell that your heart is developing problems because your heart sounds (that he can hear in his stethoscope) change. When the doctor puts his hand on the front of your chest, he feels a thumping at the place where your heart beats against the chest wall. As your heart fails, that thumping is felt farther away from the center of your chest, indicating that your heart is getting larger.

A number of signs and symptoms suggest that heart failure has appeared. These are discussed in the next section, "Noticing the telltale signs."

Noticing the telltale signs

The most common symptom of heart failure is difficulty breathing, known as *dyspnea.* At first, breathing is only difficult during exercise. As the heart failure increases, however, the individual has difficulty breathing when she's resting, too. People without heart failure may get short of breath with exercise, too, but only after exercising at least for a few minutes or so. People whose hearts are failing have difficulty breathing at the onset of exercising.

The reason that this symptom develops is that the blood vessels of the failing heart become congested with blood — sometimes even leaking into the lung tissue. The lungs, ordinarily light and filled with air, become much heavier. The diaphragm and the other muscles of respiration have a much harder time pushing air out and pulling it in. They become fatigued, and this is felt as shortness of breath.

As the lungs fill with fluid, the patient is unable to lie down flat without raising his head. When flat, more blood pools in the lungs making breathing even more difficult. The patient may need to sleep on several pillows and should his head fall off the pillows, he may have a coughing spell. This symptom is *orthopnea,* and improves when the patient sits up or raises his head.

Sometimes a severe coughing spell and shortness of breath that can't be relieved just by sitting up or raising the head can awaken the patient. This can be a terrifying experience because the patient can't catch his breath. This is *paroxysmal nocturnal dyspnea.* It's associated with an abundance of fluid in the lung tissue where it doesn't belong.

Symptoms as severe as those felt in the condition of paroxysmal nocturnal dyspnea require a call to 911 and emergency room treatment.

Other signs and symptoms of heart failure that are less specific include:

- Fatigue and weakness
- Confused mental state due to poor blood flow to the brain

Severe shortness of breath, mental confusion, severe fatigue, or the new onset of chest pain require a visit to your doctor.

What the doctor looks for

The following list presents some of the signs and symptoms that the doctor looks for when he suspects that heart failure is present. You can find many of these for yourself if you have heart failure or have a loved one with heart failure.

- **Swollen legs:** The legs swell because water is in the tissues, a condition called *edema,* which leaves a dent when the finger pushes into the skin.
- **Large liver:** A tender, large liver fills with fluid.
- **Jaundice:** Yellow eyes and yellow skin characterize this condition. The yellowing is a result of severe liver damage due to fluid in the liver.
- **Off-beat heart sounds:** Your doctor hears abnormal heart sounds with his stethoscope.
- **Rales:** These crackling sounds in the lungs indicate the presence of fluid in the lung tissue.
- **Swollen abdomen:** The abdomen swells because of fluid in the abdominal cavity.
- **Decreased urine flow:** Due to diminished blood flow to the kidneys, the body's normal production of urine decreases.
- **Cold and pale limbs:** Arms and legs are cold and pale because of poor blood flow.

As you can tell, this is a description of a very sick individual. You don't want this to be what you see in the mirror some day. Start following the recommendations in Part III right away to lower your blood pressure and decrease your chances of developing heart failure.

A chest X-ray and an electrocardiogram (EKG) can help your doctor see just how severe the heart failure is. These standard tests are done for most types of heart disease and will be done if you have heart failure.

- **Chest X-ray:** This indicates the size of the heart and the presence and extent of fluid in the lungs. Often the veins in the chest are seen in the X-ray. The blood that's backing up enlarges these veins.
- **Electrocardiogram:** This may show changes that indicate that the heart is enlarged, but often other testing shows more.

JARGON ALERT

Ejection fraction — What's your function?

Assessing the *ejection fraction* is one of the best ways to measure your heart function. The *ejection fraction* is the ratio of the amount of blood that's pushed out of the heart with each beat, called the *stroke volume,* divided by the amount of blood within the large chamber of the heart (the left ventricle) when it's completely full, the *end diastolic volume.* If the ejection fraction is low, it means that a significant fraction of the blood in the left ventricle is left inside the heart with each beat, suggesting an inefficient (failing) heart. These volumes can be determined by an ultrasound study that uses the different echo properties of blood and heart tissue to produce a picture of the heart at rest (end diastolic volume) or when pumping (end systolic volume). The amount of blood at rest minus the amount after pumping, divided by the amount at rest, gives the ejection fraction. Alternately, an X-ray study can provide the same information.

Measurements while the patient is exercising may be even more helpful because this is the time when the heart is being maximally stressed. While nonstressed values may be normal, the patient may show evidence of significant heart failure when the heart is stressed.

Treating heart failure

After heart failure is diagnosed, it's up to your doctor to give you the information and the drugs that you need to manage the condition. This is a complicated process and won't be discussed in detail here. (See *Healthy Heart For Dummies* by James M. Rippe, MD [Wiley] for more information on this treatment.) However, like all illness, successful treatment depends on your willingness to follow the doctor's recommendations. Some of your doctor's instructions and treatments may include the following:

✔ Significant reduction in salt intake, not just to lower blood pressure but even more to prevent water retention associated with increased salt

✔ Use of certain medications including

- One of a category of drugs called ACE inhibitors (see Chapter 13) to help lower blood pressure and reduce salt and water retention early in the development of heart failure

- Diuretics to eliminate salt and water through the kidneys

- Vasodilators to open the arteries

- Digitalis, a drug that increases the heart muscle's ability to contract

- Restriction of activity to give the heart a rest
- Weight loss to reduce the work of the heart
- Reduction of fluid intake

Avoiding the Risk Factors

Uncontrolled high blood pressure, by itself, makes both heart failure and heart attacks much more difficult to manage. Should they occur, controlling the high blood pressure is an early step toward managing these complications.

You can avoid or eliminate some risk factors, and some factors you can't avoid. Doing everything possible to avoid those you can helps to prevent these complications of high blood pressure and minimize their impact should they occur. The major risk factor that you can't change is a family history of early heart disease. Your choices, however, can affect the remaining factors. In this section, I want to point out how prevalent these risk factors remain and how much of a role they continue to play in the occurrence of these complications of high blood pressure and their prognosis when they do occur.

High cholesterol

Half of the U.S. adult population has abnormally high cholesterol levels. These statistics are similar for the United Kingdom, Australia and New Zealand. For a breakdown of the various ethnic populations, the rates are

- **Caucasian:** 52 percent of men and 49 percent of women
- **African American:** 45 percent of men and 46 percent of women
- **Hispanic:** 53 percent of men and 48 percent of women
- **Native American:** 38 percent of men and 37 percent of women

Looking at these numbers, it's astonishing that we don't see far more complications, especially heart attacks in association with high blood pressure. High cholesterol is treatable. The dietary changes recommended in Chapter 9 along with the exercise recommendations of Chapter 12 take care of most of it. High cholesterol that doesn't respond to diet and exercise is easily managed by a group of drugs called "statins," a powerful group of cholesterol-lowering drugs.

Find out the level of your cholesterol and bring it down. The lower your cholesterol, the better.

Tobacco use

In many ways, tobacco use is a greater problem than high cholesterol. The most important reason is that you're addicted to cigarettes, but you're not addicted to fat. Breaking the smoking habit is difficult but definitely worth doing.

About a quarter of the U.S. population is addicted to cigarette smoking. The ethnic breakdown is

- **Caucasian:** 26 percent of men and 24 percent of women smoke
- **African American:** 29 percent of men and 21 percent of women smoke
- **Hispanic:** 25 percent of men and 13 percent of women smoke
- **Native American:** 42 percent of men and 38 percent of women smoke

Just how many men and women continue to commit slow suicide is astonishing. Even more astonishing is the rate of cigarette smoking among young people who are very much aware of the statistics that relate cigarettes not only to heart disease, but to lung cancer, emphysema, and many other cancers.

In Chapter 11, I provide everything that's known about how to stop smoking — one of the most difficult tasks you may ever face. In terms of the benefits to your health, nothing you do can be of greater value.

Controlling diabetes

Now, more than 16 million Americans have diabetes. Heart attacks remain the most frequent cause of death among diabetics. Heart attacks are responsible for two-thirds of all deaths among diabetics. When they have heart attacks, they tend to be more complicated than a heart attack in a nondiabetic. The extensive nature of the atherosclerotic plaque (areas of obstruction in blood vessels) in diabetics results in a poor response to PTCA and the need for CABG when angina or a heart attack occurs.

The prognosis is less pessimistic when the diabetes is brought under control. This means keeping the blood glucose (sugar) as close to the normal range as possible (between 80 and 120 milligrams of glucose per deciliter of blood) and keeping the hemoglobin A1c, a test for long-term diabetic control, under 7 percent of the total hemoglobin.

Diabetes is diagnosed when the blood glucose is 126 milligrams per deciliter (mg/dL) on two or more occasions in the fasting state or 200 mg/dL in a random blood glucose on two or more occasions. The problem is that the increased risk of heart disease doesn't start when the blood glucose is over 126 fasting or 200 random. Between 110 and 126 in the fasting state or 140 and 200 at random, the patient is said to have impaired fasting glucose or impaired glucose tolerance. The increased risk of heart disease associated with the blood glucose is present at these levels of blood glucose as well. The number of people with these conditions isn't small. The statistics just for impaired fasting glucose are

✔ **Caucasian:** 9 percent of men and 5 percent of women

✔ **African American:** 3 percent of men and 5 percent of women

✔ **Hispanic:** 12 percent of men and 7 percent of women

The solution is to keep your weight down, get plenty of exercise, avoid fats, and keep your blood glucose under 110 fasting or 140 random. That keeps your heart risk at a minimum.

Lack of physical activity

Lack of physical activity has clearly been shown to be a risk factor for heart disease. Many people do work that requires little physical activity and exercise is needed during leisure time. This isn't happening, however. The following percentages show the populations that are sedentary:

✔ **Caucasian:** 33 percent of men and 39 percent of women

✔ **African American:** 46 percent of men and 57 percent of women

✔ **Hispanic:** 50 percent of men and 57 percent of women

Anyone who says that Americans are on the move hasn't looked at these numbers. Chapter 12 tells you how to get going and keep going. The farther you walk, the longer you live. It's as simple as that.

Chapter 6

Protecting Your Kidneys

● ●

In This Chapter

▶ Cleaning house: Your kidneys' filtering systems

▶ Finding out how kidneys affect high blood pressure

▶ Discovering how high blood pressure impairs renal function

▶ Treating end-stage renal disease and malignant high blood pressure

● ●

*A*lthough I discuss how high blood pressure affects the heart, kidneys, and brain in three separate chapters, this doesn't mean that individuals with high blood pressure develop one or the other disease — heart disease *or* kidney disease *or* a brain attack — separately. All these complications progress at the same time, and uncontrolled high blood pressure triggers the development of heart disease, kidney disease, and a brain attack all at the same time. Other factors may prevent a heart attack or brain attack (such as taking aspirin), allowing kidney disease to dominate the picture, or a patient may have only two complications at the same time for some other reason. Still, you can prevent all these complications if you control your blood pressure.

This chapter discusses the kidney and how high blood pressure damages the kidney — how it occurs, how it proceeds, and how it leads to end-stage renal disease if unchecked. If you read this whole chapter, I expect that you'll have the same great appreciation for your kidneys that I have for mine. You may even raise a glass of water and toast them!

Although efforts to reduce high blood pressure have paid huge dividends in terms of reducing heart disease and stroke, this isn't true for end-stage renal disease. This is probably because controlling the blood pressure sufficiently and for long enough simply isn't happening.

REMEMBER

Don't accept a diagnosis of high blood pressure until multiple high readings are found, and even then, measure your blood pressure at home with a reliable monitor (see Chapter 2) both to confirm the diagnosis and to follow your response to treatment. After high blood pressure is verified, it's usually persistent. However, especially when lifestyle changes are made, high blood pressure may improve even if some damage is permanent.

Looking at Your Kidneys

Your body has two kidneys, each weighing about six ounces, less than half of 1 percent of the body's total weight. Each kidney is about four inches tall, two inches wide, and one inch thick. Their position in your abdomen is shown in Figure 6-1.

Blood enters the kidneys through the large *renal arteries*. The *renal cortex* is the kidney's outer shell, containing blood vessels and urine tubes. The *renal pyramids* contain the urine tubes and specialized tissue that permits fine-tuning of the various substances that leave the kidneys in the urine. Figure 6-2 shows an inside view of the kidney's major parts.

Focusing in on the filtering function

Your kidneys are truly amazing. The digestive tract only takes out the waste that goes through the digestive tract, but the kidneys filter the blood, which acts much like a cargo carrier, dropping off nutrients and picking up waste from all the cells everywhere in your body. The blood carries waste from the cells to your body's waste-disposal headquarters — the kidneys. Separating out the recyclable material from the trash that needs to pass on to the bladder and out the urethra, the kidneys filter out what can be reused from what needs to be passed off in the form of urine.

Your kidneys filter an enormous amount of blood every minute, namely one and one-half quarts. They don't allow blood cells (such as your red blood cells and white blood cells) and large chemical compounds to pass through the filter, but everything else, including the toxins (waste products of normal metabolism) is filtered. After moving through the kidney filtering process, the kidneys reabsorb the recyclable materials — 99 percent of the desired water, sodium, and other key body elements — back into the body. A little water carries the toxins to the bladder as urine; then the urine passes out of the body through the urethra.

The process requires pressure to force the liquid part of the blood through, so the kidney has a built-in mechanism in the form of the renin-angiotensin-aldosterone system (see Chapter 4) that maintains the necessary level of blood pressure should it decline. Too much pressure for too much time causes damage. If the damage proceeds, the result is end-stage renal disease. If a patient has end-stage renal disease, his kidneys can't filter the blood and eliminate toxins without the help of dialysis or transplantation. (For more on dialysis and kidney transplants, see the "Coping with End-Stage Renal Disease" section later in this chapter.)

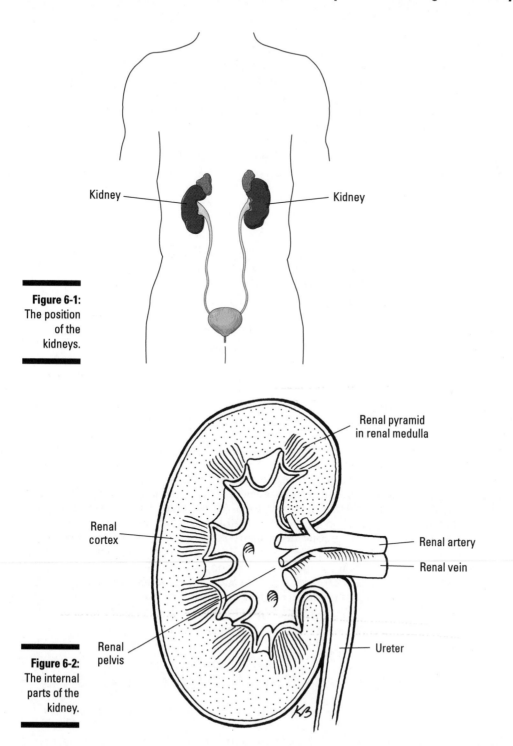

Figure 6-1:
The position
of the
kidneys.

Figure 6-2:
The internal
parts of the
kidney.

The blood makes its way through smaller and smaller arteries. Eventually, the arteries branch into capillaries, the human body's smallest blood vessels, through which the liquid part of the blood with its dissolved elements, such as sodium, potassium, uric acid, and many others, can pass.

Just before passing into a capillary, blood goes through the *afferent artery,* the artery that brings blood to the *nephron,* the kidney's filtering device. Figure 6-3 shows the *nephron.* Each kidney contains 1 million nephrons. After filtering takes place, the blood goes from a capillary into the *efferent artery.*

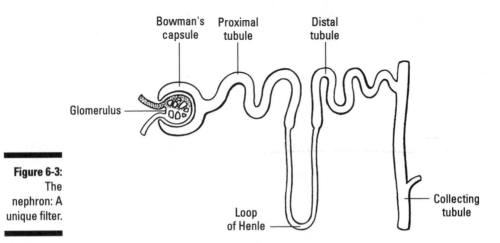

Figure 6-3:
The
nephron: A
unique filter.

The capillary network within the nephron is the *glomerulus.* The *Bowman's capsule,* a bulb that surrounds the glomerulus, receives all the water that's filtered through and begins the process of returning most of it to the bloodstream while letting all the substances that the body doesn't want out. The remaining urine ends up in the *collecting tubule,* which empties into the *renal pelvis* and then through the *ureter* to the bladder. High blood pressure, diabetes, and many other conditions destroy these nephrons and may lead to end-stage renal disease. However, it's only when about 10 percent of nephron function remains that the individual is made aware of loss of kidney function because he begins to feel sick from the failure of the kidneys to get rid of toxins. Before that, high blood pressure, anemia, and bone disease occur with loss of about 70 percent of kidney function, but the patient may not be aware of these abnormalities.

Understanding other kidney functions

In addition to filtering out and passing off your body's waste, your kidneys affect your blood pressure in other ways, too. Your kidneys also produce hormones and an important enzyme called *renin.*

Producing renin

The *juxtaglomerular cells* make and release this enzyme called *renin.* These cells are adjacent to the *afferent arterioles* — small blood vessels that carry blood to the kidney's filtering site. When the arteriole detects that the blood pressure is insufficient for filtration to take place, the juxtaglomerular cells go into action and release renin. The release of renin eventually leads to the production of angiotensin II, which has the double effect of causing

- ✔ **Blood vessel constriction:** This causes blood pressure to rise immediately.

- ✔ **Aldosterone secretion:** Blood pressure is further raised because this causes salt and water retention.

After the juxtaglomerular cells perceive a satisfactory blood pressure, they stop making more renin.

Producing hormones

Specialized cells within the kidneys produce *erythropoietin,* a hormone that stimulates the bone marrow to make more red blood cells. Whenever blood is lost or a trip to high altitude demands more oxygen, the need for red blood cells is greater, and thus the kidneys produce erythropoietin. If kidney damage occurs, the cells that make erythropoietin decline, and *anemia,* a fall in the oxygen-carrying red blood cells, develops.

Another important function of the kidneys is the production of a hormone that stimulates the uptake of calcium in the intestine. This hormone is actually the active end product of the formation of vitamin D3. The process begins in the skin where a substance is turned into vitamin D3 by the ultraviolet rays of the sun. This substance then circulates to the liver where it's converted to the next stage of active vitamin D3 production. Finally, it reaches the kidneys where the most active form is produced. When kidney function declines, highly active vitamin D3 declines. Without highly active vitamin D3, calcium isn't taken up in sufficient quantities, and poorly calcified bone is formed that's weaker than normal bone called *osteomalacia.*

Damaging the Kidney

Using renin, aldosterone, the heart muscles, and many other tools in the body, the kidney attempts to regulate the blood pressure that's felt at the glomerulus. It needs to be just high enough to push out the water and dissolved substances but not so high that it damages the glomerular cells. When this regulation fails, kidney damage begins. As kidney tissue is lost, each glomerulus that's left must do more filtering. Pressure at the glomerulus rises for this to take place, but rising pressure does more damage. So the increased pressure maintains short-term kidney function but creates more long-term damage.

Is the answer to essential high blood pressure somewhere in the kidney?

Studies show that high blood pressure damages the kidneys, but what causes the onset of high blood pressure in *essential high blood pressure* (high blood pressure for which the cause is unknown)?

Many scientists, insisting that the kidney is the source of the blood pressure elevation in essential high blood pressure, cite a study outlined in *Circulation Research* (June 1975). The study involved an experiment on rats that have hereditary high blood pressure: If a rat from a strain that's known to have normal blood pressure throughout life has its kidneys removed and receives a normal kidney from a strain that's known to develop high blood pressure later in life, the rat develops high blood pressure. But

when the opposite experiment is done — the rat that's prone to high blood pressure in the future has its kidneys removed and receives a normal kidney from a normal rat — high blood pressure doesn't develop. Therefore, the glitch must be somewhere in the kidney of the high blood pressure strain. Despite its normal appearance and that the kidney hasn't been subjected to high blood pressure as yet, the kidney that comes from the strain of rats with high blood pressure brings on high blood pressure. The rat study's main conclusion is that rats with hereditary high blood pressure lose the ability to excrete salt from their body at a young age. Salt retention leads to water retention and a subsequent rise in blood pressure.

Plenty of experimental evidence suggests that higher pressure in the glomerulus damages the kidney:

- ✔ If 90 percent of an animal's kidney is removed, the increased pressure damages the remaining glomeruli.

- ✔ When animals are fed a protein-restricted diet, which lowers glomerular blood pressure, the damage slows.

- ✔ Drugs that lower glomerular pressure, even without lowering pressure in the arm, slow the onset of damage.

- ✔ Drugs that lower arm pressure but don't lower glomerular pressure don't protect the kidneys.

Just exactly *how* increased blood pressure in the glomeruli leads to kidney damage is unclear at this point. Current research suggests that the pressure causes production of certain chemicals that stimulate increased cell growth in the glomerulus as well as injury to normal cells. As more cells grow in the tiny space of the glomerulus, the surface through which the blood can be filtered becomes less and less. *Endothelial cells* that line the inside of blood vessels make many different chemicals, including nitric oxide, an important substance that widens blood vessels, as well as chemicals that may damage blood vessels.

How untreated high blood pressure affects the kidneys

Before medications for high blood pressure control were available, a great number of subjects (people with uncontrolled high blood pressure) were studied and followed. After 15 to 25 years of no control, abnormally high levels of protein (an indication of kidney damage) were found in the urine of about 40 percent of the subjects. After this was discovered, these subjects died in about 5 years. Those subjects that had an elevation in blood urea nitrogen (evidence of kidney function loss because the kidney ordinarily eliminates this) lived about another year. A typical study can be found in the *Journal of Chronic Diseases* (January 1955) where 500 patients were followed for an average of 20 years.

After an individual is diagnosed with end-stage renal disease, life expectancy is now prolonged due in part to dialysis and kidney transplantation. Currently, about 10 percent of deaths associated with high blood pressure are due to kidney failure.

Many researchers contend that the cause of essential high blood pressure can be linked to a kidney that appears to be normal but has a diminished ability to rid the body of salt. (See the sidebar titled "Is the answer to essential high blood pressure somewhere in the kidney?" sidebar in this chapter.) This scientific perspective is further supported by the fact that a society that consumes salt in large quantities has a high incidence of high blood pressure. Chapter 10 describes the close connection between salt and high blood pressure in greater detail.

Managing Malignant High Blood Pressure

Malignant high blood pressure (often found in smokers and in young African American males) affects about 1 percent of people with high blood pressure. It refers to severely high blood pressure with a diastolic reading often greater than 150 mm Hg along with evidence of severe complications including:

✔ Severe eye damage, including

- **Papilledema:** Swelling of the optic disc, the place where the nerve enters the eye from the brain

- **Exudates:** Also called "white spots," release of fluids that are opaque in front of the retina and bleeding

- **Blindness**

✔ Progressive damage to the brain that may manifest itself as headaches to start with. Next, the individual with malignant high blood pressure may become confused and finally lapse into a coma.

✔ Rapid development of partial or total loss of kidney function

✔ Nausea and vomiting

Dramatically elevated blood pressure isn't enough to make a malignant high blood pressure diagnosis. People with the same high blood pressure reading may not have the condition. The symptoms in the preceding list are necessary to make the diagnosis.

A doctor must treat malignant high blood pressure in a hospital setting because it's a medical emergency. The patient may not have had a diagnosis of high blood pressure in the past. He may appear confused and have evidence of no remaining kidney function as well as heart failure. (A physical exam should disclose the high blood pressure as well as the poor mental functioning.) When the doctor looks in the patient's eyes, she sees swelling of the optic disc, bleeding that can be small dots or flame-shaped hemorrhages and spasm of the arteries within the eye.

The exact cause of malignant high blood pressure is unclear. Malignant high blood pressure may be the direct result of poor blood pressure control. The blood pressure is allowed to rise to this dangerous level. Additional explanations include the production of chemicals by damaged kidneys. These chemicals further damage the kidney and cause contraction of blood vessels, thus raising the blood pressure. Other chemicals that usually widen blood vessels may be suppressed.

Causes of secondary high blood pressure (see Chapter 4), especially *renal artery stenosis,* also trigger malignant high blood pressure in as many as one third of cases.

In the days before 1950 or so, when treatment for high blood pressure wasn't available, the majority of these patients were dead within six months. Now that effective treatment is available, the response to treatment depends on how much irreversible kidney damage has taken place. The treatment consists of lowering the blood pressure. If the kidney damage is minimal, then more than 90 percent of patients are alive after five years. Even among those with kidney damage, the survival is about 65 percent after five years. If these patients don't have a fatal heart attack, the eventual cause of death in these patients is end-stage renal disease, particularly if their kidneys show signs of damage.

Coping with End-Stage Renal Disease

End-stage renal disease (ESRD), also known as *chronic renal failure,* is loss of at least 90 percent of kidney function. The kidneys can't perform their primary function — waste removal. Thus, waste and excess fluid (that would normally be passed through the urethra and out of the body) builds up within the body. To continue living, the patient requires a kidney transplant or dialysis as explained later in this chapter.

High blood pressure, diabetes, and many other conditions that destroy the filtering nephrons can lead to ESRD. However, individuals who are losing their kidney function are usually unaware of it until they begin to feel sick, and often, they don't start to feel sick until 90 percent of their kidneys' ability to get rid of toxins fails. Before that, with about 70 percent of kidney function lost, high blood pressure, anemia, and bone disease can occur. But still, the individual may be unaware of these abnormalities.

Although efforts to reduce high blood pressure have paid huge dividends, such as a reduction in the rate of heart disease (see Chapter 5) and brain attacks (see Chapter 7), this isn't true for ESRD. This is probably because, throughout the world, high blood pressure isn't being controlled sufficiently and for long enough.

Whether high blood pressure is untreated or inadequately treated, the result is much the same: ESRD if the patient hasn't already died of heart disease or a brain attack.

Currently, around 300,000 people in the United States are being treated for ESRD and the number rises 10 percent each year. About half of those with ESRD are men. About two-thirds are Caucasian, and about one-third of the population is African American. The largest group is between 45 and 64 years of age. Almost a quarter of those with ESRD die each year. The cost of caring for them is 16 billion dollars each year.

The most common reason for ESRD is currently diabetes (33 percent of the time). The second most common cause is high blood pressure (25 percent of the time). Internal diseases of the kidney account for the rest.

The person with untreated ESRD is very ill. Symptoms affect the entire body and include the following:

- ✔ Fatigue and weakness
- ✔ Easy bruising

- ✔ Itchy skin
- ✔ A metallic taste in the mouth
- ✔ Breath that smells of urine
- ✔ Shortness of breath (even while sitting still and more with minimal activity)
- ✔ Nausea and vomiting
- ✔ Impotency
- ✔ Frequent urination that interrupts sleep
- ✔ Cramping and spasms in the legs (especially at night while trying to sleep)
- ✔ Irritability
- ✔ Unconsciousness

These signs and symptoms subside after treatment begins. Whether the kidneys fail because of high blood pressure, diabetes, or some other cause, the treatment at that stage, as far as the kidneys are concerned, is the same: dialysis or kidney transplantation.

The choices for the treatment of ESRD have their pluses and minuses. Ample financial resources are available for all the choices because the federal government as well as private insurance pays for most of the treatment cost. You needn't worry about paying for your care.

Lifesaving dialysis

If the kidneys fail, as in the case of ESRD, then the kidneys can't filter out the body's waste and eliminate it. As described in the "How untreated high blood pressure affects the kidneys" sidebar in this chapter, if the blood pressure is left alone and uncontrolled, an individual with ESRD couldn't expect to live much longer. So modern medicine's man-made methods of waste removal, such as *peritoneal dialysis* or *hemodialysis,* need to be employed to filter waste from the blood and rid the body of its nasty toxins.

Peritoneal dialysis

If you have ESRD, you may need peritoneal dialysis. During peritoneal dialysis, a quantity of fluid is placed in your abdomen, the body's toxins enter the fluid, and the fluid flows out. Peritoneal dialysis takes advantage of the fact that the abdominal cavity is lined with the *peritoneum,* a membrane that can act as a filter. The peritoneum prevents the passage of larger elements of the blood, such as blood cells and protein, but allows the liquid part of the blood with all its dissolved substances to pass through.

A *dialysate,* a salt-and-sugar solution, is put into the abdominal cavity through a permanent catheter that must be placed by a surgeon. Body wastes enter the dialysate solution because of their high concentration in the body. The dialysate is then drained out, along with the unwanted wastes, through the catheter. Each cycle of putting in and removing dialysate is an *exchange.* Figure 6-4 shows how peritoneal dialysis is performed.

Peritoneal dialysis is usually done at home and is much more successful if several exchanges are done per day rather than one. Three types of peritoneal dialysis can be done:

- ✔ **Continuous ambulatory peritoneal dialysis** uses gravity to fill and empty the abdomen. Usually, three to four exchanges need to be made during daytime and one during sleep.

- ✔ **Continuous cycler-assisted peritoneal dialysis** uses a machine to fill and remove the dialysate from the abdomen, especially during the night to make the overnight dialysis more efficient. Three to five exchanges are done during sleep and another takes place during daytime for a longer period. A higher concentration of sugar is used for the daytime exchange to promote more loss of wastes.

- ✔ **Nocturnal intermittent peritoneal dialysis** uses six or more nighttime exchanges with the cycler machine, so that the daytime exchange can be avoided. These patients usually have some kidney function left over because this technique isn't the most efficient.

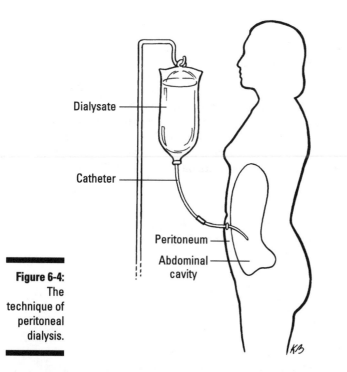

Dialysate

Catheter

Peritoneum

Abdominal cavity

Figure 6-4: The technique of peritoneal dialysis.

Testing the dialysate as well as the patient's blood and urine determines the efficiency of each exchange. Measurement of the waste products in the three fluids determines whether more dialysis needs to be done, more solution needs to be put into the abdomen, or the solution needs to have more or less sugar in it.

Home peritoneal dialysis has several pros and cons. The advantages include the following:

- ✔ The patient is in control of the treatment, so scheduling around his lifestyle is easier.
- ✔ The patient doesn't have to travel to the hospital or dialysis center.
- ✔ Dietary restrictions are minimal with the exception of protein intake.
- ✔ Carrying supplies or shipping them ahead to the destination, the patient is able to travel.
- ✔ Particularly if the patient is doing nocturnal intermittent peritoneal dialysis, the patient may exercise.

The disadvantages include

- ✔ Failure to perform the dialysis at times is common and the patient gets sick.
- ✔ The patient must be trained to do the dialysis.
- ✔ If you use a machine, then you need help from a partner.
- ✔ The dialysis bags and equipment require extra space in the home.
- ✔ *Peritonitis,* an infection of the peritoneal cavity, is a common complication of peritoneal dialysis.

Peritonitis raises body temperature. The abdomen may be tender and swell, and the patient may be nauseated and vomit. The dialysate becomes cloudy instead of clear, and bacteria may grow out from it. If you notice these symptoms, see your doctor right away. Peritonitis is treatable and usually responds well to antibiotics. However, it sometimes recurs, and the bacteria infects the catheter. Then a new catheter needs to replace the infected one.

The success of peritoneal dialysis depends on how much dialysate can be placed into the abdominal cavity and how rapidly the wastes pass into the dialysate. Some people can't use peritoneal dialysis because their peritoneum doesn't allow sufficient rapid passage of body fluids. In this case, hemodialysis may be the preferred method of treating ESRD.

Hemodialysis

During hemodialysis, your blood circulates through a dialysis machine called a *dialyzer.* The blood leaves your body and goes into the dialyzer that removes the toxins and returns the cleansed blood to you.

A surgeon performs a minor operation in which an artery and a vein are connected to form an arteriovenous *fistula* (an abnormal connection). This allows for a large blood flow. The fistula heals in a month or so, and needles can then be placed in the artery (to deliver blood to the machine) and the vein (to return blood to the body).

The blood from the artery enters the dialyzer where it passes through filters that again mimic the glomerulus. Wastes are removed while normal body components are retained or returned to the blood. The blood then returns to the body through the needle into the vein. Figure 6-5 shows how hemodialysis is done.

Hemodialysis, like peritoneal dialysis, has its share of advantages and disadvantages. Advantages include

✔ It can be done at home or at a dialysis center or within the hospital.

- Performing the treatment at home allows you to set your own schedule as long as you do it according to your doctor's recommendations.

- Taking treatment at a hospital ensures that professional help is available in case it's needed. Also, hemodialysis patients often enjoy being in the company of other patients with similar problems because it's usually done in a group at a center.

✔ Hemodialysis is usually performed three times per week for two to four hours, considerably less time than peritoneal dialysis.

Disadvantages include

✔ You must follow a fairly careful diet and avoid fluids, salt, foods that contain phosphorus, such as milk, cheese, and chocolate, and foods that contain potassium, such as citrus and tomatoes.

✔ Taking treatment away from home requires you to make regular trips to and from the hospital.

✔ The dialyzer and equipment takes up plenty of space in your home.

✔ You must be trained to administer and monitor home hemodialysis. For example, you need to know how to clamp off the needles if bleeding occurs. You also have to be vigilant about caring for the fistula or infection may occur.

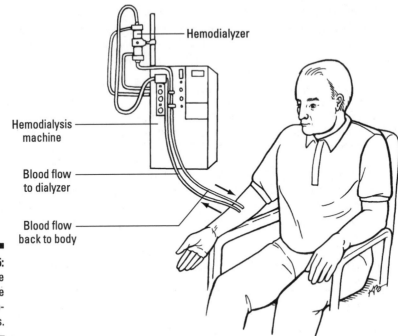

Hemodialyzer

Hemodialysis machine

Blood flow to dialyzer

Blood flow back to body

Figure 6-5:
The technique of hemo-dialysis.

Kidney transplantation

If possible, transplantation is the best answer to ESRD. You end up with a new, healthy kidney that performs like your old kidneys before they failed.

When you have a kidney transplantation, you get a new kidney from a live related donor or from a donor who has recently passed away. If the kidney comes from a relative, the surgery can be done immediately. If the kidney comes from a donor who has recently passed away, your name goes on a waiting list, and you must wait your turn. The kidney is placed in your body as shown in Figure 6-6 during surgery that takes three to six hours followed by a hospitalization of up to two weeks. The failed kidneys are usually left in, unless they're infected or causing high blood pressure. As the figure shows, the ureter is transplanted as well.

Eighty percent of transplanted kidneys, whether from family members or from unknown donors, still function after a year. On an average, kidneys from living donors survive 15 years, and kidneys from donors who've recently died last 10 years.

Kidney transplantation is a long-term solution with significant advantages including

✔ Patients feel as normal as they did before they became sick.

✔ No dialysis is necessary as long as the kidney continues to function.

✔ You only need to follow a few dietary restrictions.

Like all the treatment, however, disadvantages exist:

✔ Major surgery is required.

✔ Few kidneys are available. So if the person has to wait for a donor, it may be a long wait. Meanwhile, dialysis has to be done.

✔ Some transplants fail, and a second transplant is needed.

✔ Drugs, such as *immunosuppressants,* must be taken for a lifetime to prevent your body from rejecting the transplanted kidney. These drugs have side effects, such as the promotion of diabetes and the weakening of your immune system (making infection more likely).

✔ The drugs or rejection of the new kidney may be responsible for high blood pressure (present in up to 90 percent of transplant survivors), which can further damage the new kidney.

✔ Due to health reasons, only half of the patients on dialysis are appropriate for a transplant.

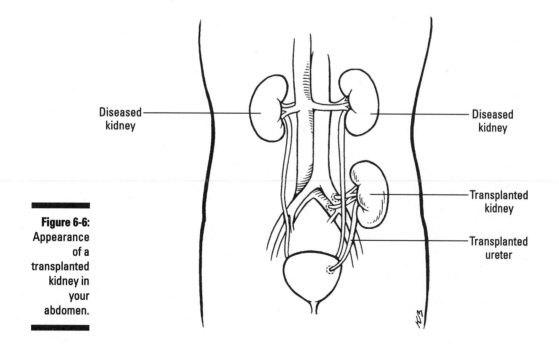

Figure 6-6:
Appearance
of a
transplanted
kidney in
your
abdomen.

Diseased kidney

Diseased kidney

Transplanted kidney

Transplanted ureter

Chapter 7

Guarding Your Brain from High Blood Pressure

• •

In This Chapter

▶ Understanding what precipitates a brain attack

▶ Finding out about the different types of brain attack

▶ Discovering how and why high blood pressure factors in

▶ Knowing the signs and symptoms

▶ Testing, treating, and getting help for the brain attack survivor

• •

*A*nnually, at least 5 million people die from brain attacks (the term I prefer over "stroke" because it's similar to a "heart attack"), and 15 million more survive it throughout the world. But brain attack survivors may live out the rest of their lives as dependents — unable to speak coherently and/or confined to a wheelchair because of the paralysis that results.

In the United States, 600,000 people have brain attacks each year and 160,000 die. The rest may suffer serious disability. Seventy percent live without the assistance of others, but 30 percent are permanently disabled. A brain attack isn't necessarily a disease of the elderly because 28 percent of the new cases are in people under age 65. In the United States, 4 million brain attack survivors have some degree of disability. In Japan, the incidence of brain attacks is rising after falling for many years. In Eastern Europe and countries of the Russian Federation, the incidence is rising, and many more brain attacks are fatal as compared to more advanced countries, such as the United States, Canada, and Western Europe.

A *brain attack,* also known as a *cerebrovascular accident* or *stroke,* occurs when blood flow to a part of the brain is cut off. Depending on the severity of the attack, victims often suffer from impaired vision and speech, convulsions, paralysis, and coma. The higher the blood pressure, the greater the likelihood of a brain attack.

Brain attacks don't favor any particular group, such as the poor or the rich, the famous or the unknown. Perhaps one of the most famous people to suffer a brain attack was U.S. President Franklin Delano Roosevelt. In 1945, as World War II was coming to a close, President Roosevelt died within a few hours of a brain attack at the age of 63 after years of poorly treated high blood pressure. The famous nineteenth-century French bacteriologist, Louis Pasteur, on the other hand, suffered a brain attack at age 46 that left him paralyzed on the left side. Yet Pasteur — making medical history and discovering, among other things, several bacteria that are responsible for the spread of infectious disease — did his best work during the next 25 years of his life.

In this chapter, you find out about the cause of brain attacks, the warning signs that predict a brain attack, and signs that a brain attack is taking place. You can discover the value of early diagnosis and early treatment. And you can find out about dealing with a brain attack survivor who now needs rehabilitation. Make sure that you make use of all the information in this chapter so that this devastating complication never makes your life miserable.

Just because I'm separating my discussion of high blood pressure and the brain from the heart (see Chapter 5) and the kidneys (see Chapter 6), doesn't mean that you'll develop brain damage from high blood pressure separate from heart disease or kidney failure. High blood pressure — the silent killer — tends to work its way on various parts of the body simultaneously. So you may discover that you have problems in all three areas all at the same time as a result of uncontrolled high blood pressure.

Understanding the Causes of Brain Attacks

The belief that brain attacks were random events, like bolts of lightning, persisted into the twentieth century along with the term *apoplexy,* coming from a Greek word meaning "to be thunderstruck." Apoplexy was the word that folks used back then to refer to a brain attack. Considered unpreventable, a brain attack was thought of as an accident, which explains the term *cerebrovascular accident.* This is clearly not the case, however, as you'll discover.

Brain attacks, perhaps more than heart attacks and kidney failure, are preventable.

Progress in the treatment of high blood pressure between 1960 and 1990 made this complication of high blood pressure less common. More recently, however, the prevention of brain attacks has slowed down. Even with the reduction in the incidence of brain attacks, it remains the third leading cause of death after heart attacks and cancer.

Although the correlation between high blood pressure and brain attacks is unmistakable, brain attacks can come about in a variety of ways. Brain attacks can result from atherosclerosis, a cerebral embolus, or a brain hemorrhage.

Atherosclerosis

Just as *atherosclerosis* (damage to the inside of arteries caused by cholesterol deposits) can affect the arteries of the heart (see Chapter 5), it can also affect the arteries leading into and within the brain. About 60 percent of all brain attacks result from *atherosclerosis,* which is characterized by fatty deposits on the inner walls of the arteries. As a result, blood flow to critical parts of the brain is diminished. If the blood flow ceases entirely, a brain attack may occur.

The blood supply to the brain has multiple sources. Figure 7-1 shows the unique circulation of blood in the brain. Left and right arteries (cerebral arteries) entering the skull in the front of the brain combine with left and right vertebral arteries entering the skull in the back of the brain to produce a circle of blood supply called the *circle of Willis* at the base of the brain. Other arteries that make up the circle are shown in the figure. If one of the arteries is blocked, blood from the other arteries can fill the circle and provide blood to all areas of the brain. So if one fails, another artery may provide the needed blood. But when several sources of blood are blocked, the brain tissue dies if the circulation isn't reopened within three hours.

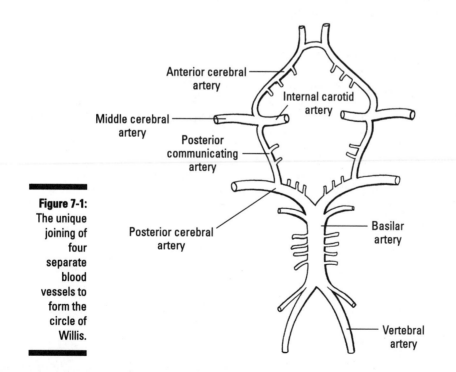

Figure 7-1:
The unique joining of four separate blood vessels to form the circle of Willis.

Cerebral embolus

Approximately 25 percent of brain attacks are due to cerebral emboli. A *cerebral embolus* is a blood clot (a solid mass of blood cells, protein, and other blood substances) or solid tissue broken off from an *atherosclerotic plaque* (an irregularity inside the artery that's the end result of a cholesterol deposit) that travels into the brain. The bloodstream carries the atherosclerotic plaque particle from its site of origin, often a large artery in the neck, into the arteries of the brain where it becomes wedged and cuts off circulation.

Blood clots usually come from the left atrium of the heart in the following manner: When the heart loses its regular beating pattern and gives way to uncoordinated twitching movements called *atrial fibrillation,* the heart's chamber (the left atrium) fails to empty out the blood that's in it completely; then the pool of blood that remains forms clots that can break off and travel via the bloodstream into the arteries of the brain.

Brain hemorrhage

Brain hemorrhage — bleeding within the brain or between the skull and the brain — accounts for the other 15 percent of brain attacks. Two-thirds of brain hemorrhages occur within the brain, and a third of brain hemorrhages occur outside the brain in the *subarachnoid space* — the technical term for the thin separation between the inside of your bony skull and the outside of your brain's fleshy gray matter.

As a result of high blood pressure or other diseases that weaken the muscular wall of the artery, one or more little pouches called an *aneurysm* may form in artery wall. With the appearance of a balloon attached to the artery, these aneurysms can burst and bleed into the brain. The brain doesn't have extra space to make room for the extra blood. Bleeding within the brain can also occur as a result of trauma to the head.

Bleeding within the subarachnoid space is usually from an aneurysm that forms inside the skull but outside the brain. If it ruptures, the blood flows around the brain, causing increased pressure and a severe headache that's often accompanied by vomiting.

Appreciating the Role of High Blood Pressure

High blood pressure is the most important factor in the development of a brain attack, and its control can prevent such an attack. High blood pressure may hasten a brain attack by

- ✔ Speeding up the development of atherosclerosis
- ✔ Promoting the thickening of the middle layer of the arteries, thus causing narrowing of the arteries and reduced blood flow into the brain
- ✔ Damaging small arteries to the point that they collapse
- ✔ Increasing the size of an aneurysm in the brain
- ✔ Causing thinning of the aneurysm to the point of rupture and hemorrhage
- ✔ Causing formation of the aneurysms in the subarachnoid space that rupture to produce a subarachnoid hemorrhage

Many clinical trials have shown that reduction of blood pressure reduces the incidence of brain attacks, no matter how high the initial blood pressure or how old the patient. All types of brain attacks are reduced, from those caused by clots to those caused by hemorrhage.

Predisposing Conditions

In addition to high blood pressure (the number one contributor to a brain attack), other predisposing conditions play an important role. These conditions (called *risk factors*) are divided into what you can't control and what you can control. Obviously, all your emphasis and energy should be directed towards those factors that you can change. However, if you have one or more unchangeable conditions, you must work even harder to minimize those factors that you can alter.

Risk factors that can't be changed

You're born with most of these uncontrollable risk factors that follow:

- ✔ **Age:** The older you get, the more you're at risk.
- ✔ **Sex:** At any age, brain attacks tend to occur more often among men than women, but more women die of brain attacks than men.

- ✔ **Family history:** If one or more of your parents and grandparents had a brain attack, then you're at risk.

- ✔ **History of brain attack:** If you're a brain attack survivor, then you're at risk for another one.

Risk factors that you can alter

This is where you can do something that can *really* make a difference. Part III is all about what you *can* do. The risk factors that are well within your power to change are

- ✔ **Arteriosclerosis:** This disease in the arteries to the brain can be treated and reopened.

- ✔ **Diabetes:** The high blood glucose of uncontrolled diabetes that's associated with high blood pressure and high cholesterol must be brought under control.

- ✔ **Atrial fibrillation:** The irregular rhythm of the heartbeat that's associated with clots that block brain arteries can be brought under control with the help of the right treatment. Ask your doctor.

- ✔ **TIA:** An acronym for transient ischemic attack (see the "Recognizing the Symptoms of an Impending Brain Attack" section later in this chapter), a TIA is a milder form of brain attack. TIA symptoms are always temporary.

- ✔ **High blood cholesterol:** Even without diabetes, cholesterol increases the risk of a brain attack.

- ✔ **Tobacco:** Smoking cigarettes or cigars or chewing tobacco causes reduction of oxygen in the blood and damages the walls of the blood vessels. Conversely, kicking your tobacco habit oxygenates the blood and decreases the likelihood of damaged blood vessels.

- ✔ **Excess weight and obesity:** Even if you're only ten pounds overweight, that excess ten pounds contributes to high blood pressure and diabetes. However, dieting and exercising can reduce your weight.

- ✔ **Lack of exercise:** A sedentary lifestyle predisposes you to a brain attack, but exercise can decrease your chances of having a brain attack drastically.

- ✔ **Birth control pills:** Especially if you're older than 30 years of age or you smoke, birth control pills can increase the incidence of blood clots that can flow to the brain. If you smoke and/or you're older than 30, you may want to discontinue the pill.

- ✔ **Illegal drugs:** Using illegal drugs, such as amphetamine, ecstasy, and cocaine, increases blood pressure and your chances of having a brain attack.

- ✔ **Alcoholic drinks:** Drinking more than two glasses of wine for men or one glass for women each night may contribute to a brain attack.

Funduscopic examination minus the fun

When a doctor looks into your eyes with the light from an ophthalmoscope (called a *fundus-copic exam*), he's observing the one area of the brain that can be seen directly. High blood pressure causes changes in the blood vessels of your eyes that are similar to those found in other small blood vessels in the brain.

The earliest change that may be seen with the ophthalmoscope is a narrowing of the arteries: The artery walls thicken and eventually the column of blood is no longer seen; then the arteries appear to be silver wires. Blood may still flow through such an artery, but it can't be seen. As the arteries thicken, nearby veins also compress, and an appearance known as *arte-riovenous* (AV) *nicking* is produced.

Your physician may see other changes in your eyes with his ophthalmoscope:

✔ The eye's major central retinal vein, which carries blood away from the retina (the

tissue that acts as a screen for sight), can close. Then vision is lost in that eye, and the appearance is one of bleeding around the back of the eye.

✔ As blood flow fails, areas of the retina die, leaving a white patchy appearance (called *cotton wool spots*).

✔ Appearing as sacs attached to arteries, aneurysms can form in the arteries of the eyes just as elsewhere in the brain due to the high blood pressure. They rarely cause hemorrhage within the eye, but if they do, it may be necessary to clot them with laser treatment.

✔ Hemorrhaging from the retina's arteries produces a flame-shaped area in the retina — a sign of out-of-control high blood pressure, also known as *malignant* or *accelerated hypertension* (discussed in Chapter 6).

If you keep these risk factors under control, you're sure to decrease the likelihood of a disabling brain attack.

Recognizing the Symptoms of an Impending Brain Attack

The symptoms of an impending brain attack come on suddenly. Don't waste a minute getting to a hospital. You may prevent much of the damage if treatment is given within the first three hours. Should you experience any of the following symptoms or should you be in the presence of another individual who is displaying any one or all of the following symptoms, don't hesitate to call an ambulance.

✔ Sudden blurred or decreased vision in one or both eyes

✔ Numbness, weakness, or paralysis of the face and/or an arm and/or a leg on one or both sides of the body

✔ Difficulty speaking or understanding

✔ Sudden dizziness, loss of balance, or an unexplained fall

✔ Difficulty swallowing

✔ Sudden headache or change in the pattern of headaches

Sometimes these symptoms may last no more than 24 hours. The condition is then called a *transient ischemic attack* (TIA), which is usually the result of reversible narrowing of certain arteries that expand over time or perhaps from small emboli that briefly interrupt blood flow and are dissolved or *bypassed* (using a blood vessel or artificial tube to go around the blockage).

One third of TIA victims eventually suffer a severe brain attack with permanent symptoms, but the other two-thirds will not. TIAs must be taken seriously, and the patient needs a doctor's evaluation to see if the cause is an atherosclerotic plaque in an artery or atrial fibrillation.

Determining the Brain Site That Loses Function

The brain is specialized so that each area performs certain functions. When a brain attack occurs, the doctor pinpoints the part of the brain that's damaged. Figure 7-2 shows the location of the various functions.

As you can see, loss of blood supply to specific areas of the brain can result in the loss of a specific function and consequent signs and symptoms. Because the right side of the brain controls the left side of the body and because the nerves cross over, careful mapping of the loss of function can determine the area of the brain that's damaged. For example, paralysis of the left leg means that the right brain leg control area is knocked out.

Some functions, such as memory, however, aren't found on both sides of the body, and the site of their control in the brain is only on one side or the other. If the brain attack affects the right side of the brain, for example, the victim may experience weakness or paralysis on the left side of his body as well as some of the following symptoms:

✔ Tendency to be impulsive or disorganized

✔ Lack of coordination and tendency to fall

✔ Inability to remember because of memory loss

✔ Lack of insight and judgment

If the brain attack occurs on the left side of your brain, you may experience right-sided weakness or paralysis as well as some difficulty communicating.

Although specific sites in the brain affect a corresponding bodily function, which arteries affect that specific site in the brain isn't as easily understood or located. This is because of the overabundance of cross circulation in the brain. Therefore, careful mapping of the function loss can determine the area of the brain that's affected, but determining the source of the impairment, such as an aneurysm within an artery that feeds the brain, may be extremely difficult.

Other symptoms may follow a brain attack that aren't necessarily particular to brain cell loss on one side or the other. For example, the brain attack survivor may be depressed or may suffer mood swings — suddenly bursting into laughter for no apparent reason. Because the person doesn't see or think as she did before, her perceptions are altered. Because one side of the body is weaker and vision on that side may be poorer, the individual may lose awareness of what goes on around that side of her body. She tends to bump into things with that side.

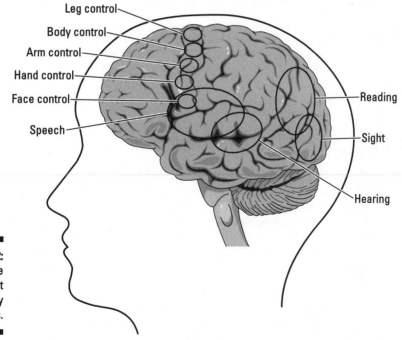

Figure 7-2:
Sites in the brain that control body functions.

Testing to Locate the Trouble Spot

The doctor may need to perform various sophisticated tests to clarify where in the brain that damage has occurred and why. The following list describes a few of the tests that your doctor may perform:

- **Computerized axial tomography** (commonly known as a CAT scan) or **magnetic resonance imaging** (MRI) can pinpoint the location of dead brain cells. These are specialized X-ray studies that can examine minute areas of the brain. They can also differentiate between a TIA and a hemorrhage. Also, the MRI can look for aneurysms and malformations in the arteries and veins that could eventually cause hemorrhage. The patient's head is placed within a circular machine while the X-rays are taken from different angles. It's painless!

- An **electroencephalogram** (EEG), a test of electrical activity in the brain, can indicate if and where the brain continues to function. An EEG is often used to determine whether some unconscious person is brain dead after a brain attack, so a ventilator (to help the victim breathe) can be continued or disconnected. It's done by applying electrodes directly onto the scalp surface — the procedure isn't painful.

- **Doppler ultrasound** tests evaluate blood flow in an artery. Sound waves are directed to the artery, usually in the neck in this case. The frequency of the returning sound indicates whether blood is flowing slowly or normally.

- **Digital subtraction angiography** (DSA) involves the injection of a dye directly into the brain's circulation; then X-rays are taken. A DSA can pinpoint the brain's blood vessels that are prohibiting normal circulation of the blood.

Treating the Brain Attack

When a brain attack occurs, usually an area called the *ischemic core* in the brain has suffered a permanent loss of brain cells. A larger area around that ischemic core called the *ischemic penumbra* is still alive and can be saved with quick action using a *tissue plasminogen activator* (tPA) or another clot-dissolving drug to break up any clot or obstruction to the flow of blood. It must be done within the first three hours after the brain attack to really benefit the brain and prevent more tissue loss.

Obviously, a tPA can't be used in a hemorrhagic brain attack because a hemorrhagic brain attack doesn't involve blood clots that need breaking up. Unfortunately, hemorrhage is an occasional side effect of tPAs. The hemorrhage can then bring on a brain attack.

If you have a TIA, aspirin is recommended to prevent further attacks. A drug that acts to prevent clotting called *warfarin* (also known as *coumadin*) is often prescribed if the TIAs are frequent and unstable. Warfarin is also prescribed for atrial fibrillation when clots form in the left atrium of the heart. (See the "Cerebral embolus" section earlier in this chapter.) Surgery can be done, especially if the arteries external to the brain, the carotid arteries, can be shown to be obstructed. But surgery may not cure the problem because the brain's blood supply comes from so many blood vessels. So even if surgery successfully repairs one blood vessel, one or more other blood vessels may also be obstructed. The surgery (called an *endarterectomy*) involves removing the material that's obstructing the artery.

When a bleeding aneurysm is the source of the brain attack, an attempt is made to "clip" or tie off the aneurysm so that it can't rupture and continue to bleed. Whether this "clipping" is done, depends on the location of the aneurysm. It may not be approachable without damaging important brain tissue.

Rehabilitating the Brain Attack Victim

Preventing a brain attack is so much better than having to deal with the consequences of a brain attack. Nevertheless, millions of people throughout the world have suffered brain attacks. An enormous amount of resources are available for brain attack survivors. The next few pages provide some insights into what the brain attack victim can expect after the attack and how to get help. The Internet can be a great resource and some useful sites are offered.

Current methods of treatment are excellent, and resources are so great that the vast majority of people who have suffered a brain attack can return to some level of satisfactory function in the long term.

Following the brain attack

Most people who have had a brain attack have trouble swallowing initially because the swallowing muscles and the mouth have been affected. They must often be supported with intravenous feeding until they can swallow without the food going into the trachea, the tube leading into the lungs.

It may take a month after the brain attack to determine how much function is going to return and what retraining has to take place. However, rehabilitation is begun within 24 hours of a stroke if the patient is stable enough. The patient is encouraged to move and change position often. If limbs are paralyzed, the nurse or physical therapist moves the limbs passively. The patient goes from lying in bed to sitting to standing and walking if possible.

Sex after a brain attack

You don't have to give up sex after a brain attack. Sex doesn't increase the risk of another brain attack. After you've stabilized, you can have sexual relations consistent with whatever limitations the brain attack has imposed. Sex after a brain attack is most pleasurable when the same conditions are present as before a brain attack: the right partner, the right environment, and the right feelings.

As time passes, therapists help the patient to perform the "activities of daily living," such things as bathing, shaving, brushing teeth, combing hair, and using the toilet. As these are regained, the patient begins to have confidence that his life isn't over, and that he may be able to function independently after all.

Where rehabilitation is performed

Where rehabilitation is carried out and just what's done depends on the limitations of the brain attack survivor. Several rehabilitation choices are available, and rehabilitation can take place in an inpatient rehabilitation unit if the survivor is immobile and unable to take care of himself. The inpatient rehabilitation unit has physical therapists, doctors, specialized nurses, and the best equipment for helping the patient regain self-sufficiency. Rehabilitation is carried out several hours daily, six days a week to promote restoration of function. The unit carefully analyzes the survivor's level of function and sets clear goals to be achieved at acceptable times for restoration of function.

After the survivor can move around fairly well or if the physical disabilities don't prevent a satisfactory life outside the hospital, he goes to an outpatient rehabilitation unit, returning home after treatment. This is usually at the hospital with the same doctors, nurses, and other specialists but doesn't take place on a daily basis. The program depends on the survivor's needs.

Brain attack survivors who aren't ready to go home alone but who aren't so debilitated that they need the inpatient rehabilitation unit are then sent to a nursing facility. Skilled nursing facilities perform rehabilitation while a nursing home provides mostly food and shelter along with medications as needed.

Sometimes, the physical therapist comes to a person's home because the brain attack survivor can live at home but can't be transported to the hospital. This is also an opportunity for the therapist to inspect the home and offer suggestions for protecting the patient from accidents and making activities of daily living more efficient.

Who does the rehabilitation?

The *physiatrist* is the doctor who specializes in physical medicine and rehabilitation. She completely evaluates the patient and determines the patient's physical limitations. With the help of the other rehabilitation specialists, a plan of action is drawn up. Goals and time frames are set and the plan is begun. The following list includes the titles and responsibilities of other rehabilitation specialists:

- **Rehabilitation nurse:** Trains the brain attack patient to perform the activities of daily living, including transfers from bed to chair, bathing, and controlling urination if incontinence is a problem.

- **Physical therapist:** Helps the patient to regain muscular movement. They promote the use of the affected limbs to strengthen them and the use of the unaffected limbs to compensate for loss of function. To overcome the lack of awareness of affected limbs, they use the technique of *selective sensory stimulation,* stimulating the limbs in one way or another to get the patient to be aware of them.

- **Occupational therapist:** Teaches the skills needed to perform work, whether it's cleaning the house, gardening, painting, or other crafts. They teach ways to perform tasks that require two hands, for example, to be done with one hand. They're the people who go into the home and make it safe for the patient as well as more efficient.

- **Speech-language pathologists:** Help patients who've developed *aphasia,* inability to speak properly after a brain attack, to regain speech. They also evaluate swallowing and determine the cause of a swallowing disability. After this is done, the speech-language pathologist can provide techniques to correct the problem.

- **Vocational therapist:** Helps the patient to regain useful work using their greatest strengths. They work as job counselors for the patient, informing them of their rights as disabled workers. They find suitable work depending on the patient's residual limitations.

Finding Help After a Brain Attack

Resources for the person who has suffered a brain attack are plentiful. Most of them can be located on the Internet, but because some people don't have access to the Internet, I also provide addresses so that you can get information through the mail as well.

With these resources and the amazing number of links that their Web sites point to, you should have no trouble getting any question answered. Someone else who has had the same experience or has asked the same question is always out there.

- The National Institute of Neurological Disorders and Stroke (NINDS) has a **Brain Resources and Information Network** (BRAIN). This is a huge database on every aspect of brain attacks. Of great interest are the studies that patients can enter, such as "The Use of Aspirin to Prevent Strokes" and "Vitamin Therapy for Prevention of Strokes" among many others. They have numerous publications and fact sheets that you can copy on the Internet or order. Write to BRAIN, P.O. Box 5801, Bethesda, MD 20820 or call 800-352-9424. On the Internet, go to www.ninds.nih.gov/health_and_medical/disorders/stroke.htm.

- **The American Stroke Association** is a subdivision of the American Heart Association. They feature many publications that are online or available by mail on the cause of brain attacks — the natural history, the treatment, and all kinds of publications about high blood pressure. They offer a *Stroke Connection Magazine* that provides timely articles on all aspects of brain attacks. They also answer your questions on the phone at 800-553-6321. They have a registry of over 2,000 stroke support groups. Contact the American Stroke Association at 7272 Greenville Avenue, Dallas, TX 75231; Phone: 800-242-8721; Internet: www.strokeassociation.org/Who_We_Are/who.html.

- **The National Stroke Association** calls itself the "voice for stroke." Its mission is "to reduce the incidence and impact of this life-threatening medical condition." It offers publications on the Internet and by mail on the cause, prevention, and treatment of a brain attack, and rehabilitation after a brain attack. Write to the National Stroke Association at 9707 East Easter Lane, Englewood, CO 80112; Phone: 800-787-6537; Internet: http://stroke.org/index.cfm.

- **Strokes Clubs International** offers help and experience from people with brain attacks to people with brain attacks. Write to Strokes Clubs International at 805 12th Street, Galveston, TX 77550 or call 409-762-1022.

- **The National Aphasia Association** promotes public education, research, rehabilitation and support services to assist people with aphasia and their families. It sells gifts that educate and helps to form support groups for aphasia patients. It offers many personal accounts of a brain attack and the aphasia that followed. Its page of Weblinks on aphasia would be valuable if nothing else were at the site, but it's packed with useful information. Write to the National Aphasia Association at 156 Fifth Avenue, Suite 707, New York, NY 10010 or call 800-922-4622. Find the association on the Internet at http://aphasia.org.

✔ The federal government funds the **National Rehabilitation Information Center** to serve anyone on topics concerning rehabilitation. Their database is vast and the links that they offer to sites that have more information on rehabilitation topics are outstanding. Write to the National Rehabilitation Information Center at 1010 Wayne Avenue, Suite 800, Silver Spring, MD 20910 or call 800-346-2742. Find the center on the Internet at www.naric.com.

✔ For people taking care of others, the **Family Caregiver Alliance** offers everything you need to know, not only about care giving for brain attacks but for many other medical conditions as well. It was the first organization to offer help to those caring for a loved one. Write to the Family Caregiver Alliance at 690 Market Street, Suite 600, San Francisco, CA 94104 or call 800-445-8106. Find the alliance on the Internet at www.caregiver.org/who.html.

Part III
Treating High Blood Pressure

The 5th Wave   By Rich Tennant

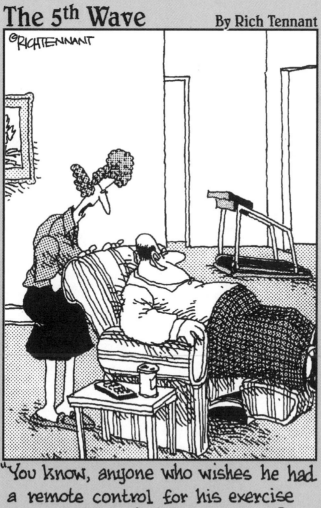

"You know, anyone who wishes he had a remote control for his exercise equipment is missing the idea of exercise equipment."

In this part . . .

Fortunately, you can treat high blood pressure in multiple ways so that it never does any damage to you. Starting with lifestyle changes and ending with drugs (only if absolutely necessary), this part gives you all the tools that you need to accomplish this. No one need ever suffer a heart attack, a brain attack, or kidney failure as a result of high blood pressure.

Chapter 8

Outlining a Successful Treatment Plan

*T*wo truths should motivate you to create a successful treatment plan for your high blood pressure:

✔ High blood pressure must be brought under control to prevent the devastating consequences of uncontrolled high blood pressure, which can damage your heart, kidneys, and brain (described in Part II).

✔ High blood pressure can be brought under control in any patient using the tools that are currently available.

Since the mid-1990s, the U.S. Centers for Disease Control has published a report card on the nation's health. Grades are given for various areas of diagnosis and treatment. A hypertension report card on the nation, based on the opinions of some of the nation's leading medical groups, was added in 1999. The results are eye opening to say the least:

✔ Healthcare professionals gave a C- grade to the overall control of high blood pressure in the United States and the nation's overall concern about the importance of treating high blood pressure.

✔ The lowest grade, a D+, went to patient understanding of high blood pressure (hence this book).

✔ A similar low D+ grade went to physician/patient communication about the topic of high blood pressure.

✔ C- was given for patient compliance with a treatment plan for high blood pressure.

✔ Another C- was given for patient satisfaction with the treatment process. It was noted that physicians spend little time with their patients on this problem; physicians don't seem sensitive to their patients' quality of life.

✔ Satisfaction with current medications received a C+. Despite the large number of available medications (see Chapter 13), satisfaction with their ease of administration, effectiveness, and side effects is low.

This performance is unacceptable. Other countries are doing no better and are generally worse. You and your physician are the ones who can turn this around. Start right now — sit down and write an outline for the elements of a successful treatment plan.

Making the Grade: Your Treatment Goal

You need to have a goal in order to know where you're going. Your particular goal depends on what your blood pressure is now. If you have normal blood pressure (less than 140/90 mm Hg), you want to keep it normal. If you already have high blood pressure, you want to lower it into the normal range and keep it there. If you already have complications of high blood pressure, you want to prevent them from progressing and even reverse them if possible.

Table 8-1 shows what category your blood pressure falls into and the recommended follow-up. (Also, see the table on blood pressure classifications in Chapter 2.)

Damage due to high blood pressure is continuous. *Target-organ damage* (damage to organs of the body from high blood pressure) doesn't start suddenly at 140/90 mm Hg. A person with normal blood pressure has more of a chance of suffering complications associated with their blood pressure than a person with optimal blood pressure. The fact that target-organ damage from high blood pressure creeps up on you slowly also means that people in the high-normal range average more medical complications than those in the normal range.

Table 8-1	Recommended Follow-up Based on Initial Blood Pressure Measurements*		
Category	*Systolic (mm Hg)*	*Diastolic (mm Hg)*	*Follow-up*
Normal	Less than 130	Less than 85	Recheck in 2 years
High normal	130–139	85–89	Recheck in 1 year; give lifestyle advice
Stage 1 HBP	140–159	90–99	Confirm in 2 months; lifestyle advice

107/65
133/79

Category	Systolic (mm Hg)	Diastolic (mm Hg)	Follow-up
Stage 2 HBP	160–179	100–109	Evaluate/refer to care within 1 month
Stage 3 HBP	180	110	Evaluate/refer to care within 7 days

Courtesy of The National Heart, Lung and Blood Institute of the National Institutes of Health in the Sixth Report of the Joint National Committee on Detection, Evaluation, and Treatment of High Blood Pressure (1997)

The National Heart, Lung and Blood Institute of the National Institutes of Health in the Sixth Report of the Joint National Committee on Detection, Evaluation, and Treatment of High Blood Pressure (1997) provides a list of important risk factors to group patients with high blood pressure for treatment. The risk factors are

✔ Diabetes

✔ Family history of heart disease

✔ High blood cholesterol

✔ More than 60 years of age

✔ Smoking

These risk factors determine exactly what stage a patient falls into when combined with whether the organs that high blood pressure affects — the so-called target organs, such as the heart, eyes, kidneys, and brain — are damaged. Target-organ damage includes the following:

✔ Angina (heart pain) or a heart attack (see Chapter 5)

✔ Enlarged heart

✔ Eye damage (see Chapter 7)

✔ Heart failure

✔ Kidney damage (see Chapter 6)

✔ Peripheral vascular disease (disease in the large blood vessels to the legs and arms)

✔ Stroke (brain attack) or transient ischemic attack (see Chapter 7)

Combining risk factors with target-organ damage, the Sixth Report of the Joint National Committee comes up with the following risk groups:

✔ **A:** No risk factors and no target-organ damage

✔ **B:** At least one risk factor not including diabetes and no target-organ damage

✓ C: Diabetes with or without other risk factors and target-organ damage

Now, based on the risk group and the level of the blood pressure, the treatment recommendations are shown in Table 8-2:

Table 8-2	Treatment Strategies Based on Risk Groups and Blood Pressure*		
Blood Pressure	**Risk Group A**	**Risk Group B**	**Risk Group C**
High-normal	Lifestyle change	Lifestyle change	Lifestyle change & drug therapy
Stage 1	Lifestyle change & 12-month trial	Lifestyle change & 6-month trial (If more than 1 risk factor is present, then drugs are prescribed.)	Lifestyle change & drug therapy
Stages 2 and 3	Lifestyle change & drug therapy	Lifestyle change & drug therapy	Lifestyle change & drug therapy

Courtesy of The National Heart, Lung and Blood Institute of the National Institutes of Health in the Sixth Report of the Joint National Committee on Detection, Evaluation, and Treatment of High Blood Pressure (1997)

According to the information in Table 8-2, people with high-normal blood pressure can lower their blood pressure with a change to their lifestyle. However, if target-organ damage is discovered in an individual with high-normal blood pressure, drugs are prescribed immediately. If you have Stage 1 high blood pressure and you have no risk factor or target-organ damage, you have 12 months to bring your blood pressure down with lifestyle change alone. If no target organ is damaged and at least one risk factor is present, you have six months to bring your blood pressure down with lifestyle change alone. Stage 1 high blood pressure requires immediate drug therapy if a target organ is damaged. In general, Stage 2 and Stage 3 high blood pressure require drug treatment along with lifestyle changes.

Consider the following examples:

✓ Say you're a 65-year-old man whose blood pressure is 145/95 mm Hg. You've never had target-organ damage. Your age (older than 60) gives you one risk factor. Because you've never had target-organ damage, you're in Risk Group B. Your blood pressure puts you in Stage 1. Where Stage 1 and Risk Group B come together, it tells you that you should try to modify your lifestyle. You try this for 6 months. If your blood pressure hasn't come down enough to put you in the high-normal range, you need to start drug therapy. If it has come down, you can continue with your lifestyle changes.

✔ Suppose you're a 55-year-old woman with diabetes whose blood pressure is 165/105 mm Hg. You have an eye disease that's associated with high blood pressure, and you smoke. The target-organ damage in your eye puts you in Risk Group C. The blood pressure is Stage 2. You must quit smoking and make some lifestyle changes to bring down your blood pressure, but you must also start drug therapy.

Determine what your blood pressure is now with the help of your physician. Discuss your risk factors and how they determine the risk group into which you fit. Then use the doctor's expertise to formulate a plan to reverse your risk factors and lower your blood pressure.

A few examples from my practice can help you to understand what you have to do.

✔ Joe Chang is a 43-year-old Chinese American who came to me because his blood pressure was elevated. Examining him, I determined that he was 5 feet and 5 inches tall and weighed 180 pounds. He didn't have diabetes or any other risk factor. He hadn't followed a diet and didn't exercise. On several different occasions, I found that his blood pressure was about 144/95 mm Hg. Based on the table of treatment strategies, I told him to begin a program of diet and exercise and referred him to a dietitian. Three months later, he had lost ten pounds and was exercising regularly. His blood pressure had fallen to 138/86 mm Hg. He has continued the program and lost an additional ten pounds with continued good blood pressure control.

✔ Elaine David, a 38-year-old mother of two children, has diabetes. She weighs 160 pounds and is 5 feet 3 inches tall. I have been following her through her two uncomplicated pregnancies. Recently, her blood pressure has measured 165/98 mm Hg. She doesn't have any other risk factors in the list in the "Making the Grade: Your Treatment Goal" section earlier in this chapter. Using the number that puts her in the higher blood pressure stage and the fact that diabetes places her in risk group C, Elaine needed to lose weight, exercise more, reduce her salt intake, and get on drug treatment. She was placed on hydrochlorothiazide 12.5 milligrams daily and propranolol was added when her blood pressure was still over 140/90 mm Hg. On this treatment, plus weight loss and exercise, her blood pressure is now 132/80 mm Hg and she feels well.

✔ Phil Sweeney was a 62-year-old, new patient. His weight was appropriate for his height. His blood pressure, however, was 175/105 mm Hg, and he had evidence of eye damage due to high blood pressure as well as an enlarged heart. On this basis, I started him on medication, asked him to continue his good diet with some salt reduction and asked him to do a little more exercise. His response has been gratifying with reduction in the size of his heart and a drop in his blood pressure to 136/88 mm Hg. He has done some meditation as well, and this seems to help. He tells me he feels like a new man.

Choosing Lifestyle Modifications

Chapters 9 through 13 of this book discuss the suggested lifestyle changes in detail. In the following section, I outline them so that you have the complete picture of the general approach to high blood pressure treatment. See Chapter 13 for a complete discussion of treating high blood pressure with medication.

Altering your lifestyle for the better

The Sixth Report of the Joint National Committee on Detection, Evaluation and Treatment of High Blood Pressure issued in 1997 recommends the following lifestyle modifications:

- Stop smoking or chewing tobacco (Chapter 11)
- Lose weight (Chapters 9 and 12)
- Limit alcohol intake (Chapter 11)
- Increase physical activity (Chapter 12)
- Reduce salt in your diet (Chapters 9 and 10)
- Maintain adequate potassium, calcium, and magnesium in your diet (Chapters 9 and 10)
- Reduce saturated fat and cholesterol in your diet (Chapter 9)

The preceding list contains no surprises with the possible exception of maintaining potassium, calcium, and magnesium. Doctors have known that these minerals help to lower blood pressure for years. Making sure that you get sufficient quantities of these minerals in your diet is wise. For extra potassium, make sure that your diet includes plenty of fruits and beans. Milk and other dairy products can provide the calcium that you need, although it's often recommended that women need to get extra calcium in supplemental form. To make sure that you're ingesting enough magnesium, increase your intake of green leafy vegetables, nuts, seeds, and whole grains.

Modify your lifestyle one step at a time. First, start cutting back or eliminating smoking or chewing tobacco because this is by far the most dangerous (see Chapter 11). Move on to reducing alcohol intake. After you've rid yourself of these habits or at least cut back dramatically, go on to strengthen your heart and body through exercise.

Pretend for a moment that your blood pressure is 140/85 mm Hg. You don't have any target-organ damage, but you have several risk factors including high cholesterol and a family history of heart disease, so lifestyle changes are in order. Your doctor warned you that you must quit your pack-a-day smoking habit, drop 20 pounds, and engage in 30 minutes of aerobic activity on a daily basis. You know that you can't just turn your sedentary lifestyle around on a dime, so you chart out a plan like the one in Table 8-3 to incorporate your doctor's advice slowly but surely over a six-month time period.

Table 8-3	Sample Plan for Lifestyle Changes		
Time Period	*Daily Smoking Limit*	*Daily Exercise*	*Weight Loss*
Week 1	Half pack		
Week 2	5 cigarettes	Walk ½ mile	
Week 3	1 cigarette	Walk ¾ mile	
Week 4	None	Walk 1 mile	
Weeks 5–8	None	Walk ½ mile & Jog ½ mile	5 lb.
Weeks 9–12	None	Walk ¼ mile & Jog ¾ mile	4 lb.
Weeks 13–16	None	Jog 1 mile	4 lb.
Weeks 17–20	None	Jog 1 mile	4 lb.
Weeks 21–24	None	Jog 1 mile	3 lb.

Plan and then chart your progress. You may want to work out a plan like the one in Table 8-3 and then keep a daily diary of how many cigarettes you actually smoke, what you eat, and how much you exercise.

TIP

To keep a health record, go on the Internet at www.lifeclinic.com. At Lifeclinic.com, you can track your blood pressure, pulse, weight, cholesterol, blood sugar, personal health records, family health records, and a health checklist.

Blood sugar Machine

As you work on each change, each new healthy habit affects many of the others. For example, increasing your level of exercise will invigorate you and increase your tolerance for stress; thus, you'll be less likely to smoke or drink alcohol when you want to relax. Similarly, the fewer cigarettes that you smoke, the easier it will for you to exercise without having to stop and catch your breath because your lung capacity will increase. These changes can also help you to lose weight as well. You may gain a few pounds as you stop smoking but the benefits of stopping smoking far outweigh (pun intended) those few pounds. Reducing the fat in your diet will help almost all the other risk factors as well. By the time you've gone through the list, you'll feel like a new person.

Tickling your funny bone

You rarely find any mention of humor and its place in the management of high blood pressure in a book about high blood pressure. This may be because it's so difficult to quantify. Scientists like to study what they can measure and the effects of humor aren't in that category. I suppose you could take two groups, subject one to humor and the other to nonhumorous experiences and measure their blood pressure before and after. That might tell you about the immediate consequences of humor but not about its long-term effects.

Laughter is good for what ails you

People such as author Norman Cousins and Joel Goodman, the head of the
Humor Project, Inc. (see more on the Internet: www.humorproject.com),
advocate humor for the management of most diseases. High blood pressure,
often associated with stress, would seem like a natural focus for the positive
effects of humor. The positive psychological and physiological effects of
laughter have been demonstrated in a variety of settings. Mirth and merri-
ment certainly reduce stress hormone production — the hormones known to
raise blood pressure.

An interesting study in the *International Journal of Cardiology* (August 2001)
indicated an inverse relationship between the tendency to find things funny
and the occurrence of coronary heart disease. A questionnaire was given to
300 people that assessed their tendency to laugh under a variety of situations
encountered in everyday life. The people with coronary heart disease were
not laughers. Those without the disease were. The results suggest that a tendency to laugh protects the heart.

Using humor in your life

The last 30 years of experience with my patients convinces me that those
who experience life with a certain degree of lightness, who are unwilling to
take life too seriously, do much better than those who don't. I carry a card
around that Dr. Joel Goodman gave me that says, "Someday we will laugh
about this. Why wait?" For most situations, it's an excellent prescription.
Laughter signifies positive things to people. It adds to feelings of closeness,
friendliness, and togetherness.

Even without definite proof of the value of humor, I recommend that you use
it as an important part of your treatment of high blood pressure. How can
you go about doing this? I recommend that you find out for yourself what
makes you laugh. Each person has a different source of amusement. Some
people like clowns; others like standup comedians. Some prefer comedians
like Eddie Murphy, while others think Woody Allen is a scream.

Find a reference book at your local library that lists movies by category such
as humor, mystery, tragedy, and so forth. Pick out a few of the top-rated comedies. You may start with *Some Like It Hot, Annie Hall, Babe, Beverly Hills Cop,*

or *Blazing Saddles. Seven Brides for Seven Brothers* and *Singin' in the Rain* may not make you laugh out loud (though they could), but you'll come away feeling much better about life in general. The old Marx Brothers comedies, Bob Hope or the newer stuff like *American Pie,* the movies of Ben Stiller or John Cusack may appeal to you. Try to see one at least once a week without fail.

Find a comedian you like and buy his or her monologues to listen to in your car. Just be careful as you drive.

My bet is that this will bring your blood pressure down. It may be a direct effect of the humor, or it may be that the humor puts you into a good mood — a mood that's good enough to take your medications consistently, stay on your diet, or do your exercise.

Like every one of the other recommendations in this chapter, turning yourself on to humor is a lifestyle change for most of us. So what if it's not backed up by the latest scientific evidence. You can't find a more pleasurable lifestyle change. I remember a quote that I read some time ago from W. H. Auden in his book, *The Dyer's Hand and Other Essays* (Faber): "Among those whom I like or admire, I can find no common denominator. But among those whom I love, I can. All of them make me laugh."

He (or she) who laughs, lasts.

Chapter 9

Eating and High Blood Pressure

● ●

In This Chapter

▶ Following a diet that lowers blood pressure

▶ Finding out how DASH can help

▶ Lowering salt intake and losing weight, too

▶ Watching your kilocalories and seeking assistance

● ●

They say that you are what you eat. When it comes to blood pressure, that statement is truer than you may realize. Weight loss with the help of a well-balanced diet and salt intake reduction can lower blood pressure. These approaches, however, haven't successfully lowered blood pressure permanently and kept it down in most patients. A new approach is needed.

In this chapter, you discover a new approach to healthy eating — the DASH diet. I explain how it developed, proved effective, and how you can use it to reduce your blood pressure, no matter what your blood pressure level is now. For those of you who want to reduce your weight for whatever reason, I provide a sensible, balanced program to help you get there. I try not to use the D (diet) word, but I encourage you to follow a sensible nutritional program.

DASHing Down Your Blood Pressure

Based on the results of studies at four major medical centers in the United States, the "Dietary Approach to Stop Hypertension" (DASH), was published in the *New England Journal of Medicine* (April 1997). All patients on the DASH diet successfully reduced their systolic and diastolic blood pressure. Table 9-1 in this chapter shows the average reduction in millimeters of mercury for the systolic blood pressure and the diastolic blood pressure for the various groups that followed the DASH diet.

Table 9-1	Average reduction in systolic (SBP) and diastolic (DBP) on the DASH diet in millimeters of mercury	
Group	**SBP**	**DBP**
African Americans	6.9	3.7
Caucasians	3.3	2.4
Established high BP	11.6	5.3
No high BP	3.5	2.2

This was achieved without special foods, food supplements, drugs, and without weekly meetings. Furthermore, it was achieved without emphasizing weight loss by reducing kilocalories, without insisting on salt intake reduction, and without demanding exercise.

Leading up to DASH

Creation of the DASH began when it was noted that vegetarians generally have lower blood pressure and a lower incidence of coronary heart disease and brain attacks (see Chapter 7) than nonvegetarians. Exactly why this was so wasn't clear. The big difference between vegetarians and nonvegetarians is that the former eat more fruits and vegetables than the latter. They also, of course, eat no meat and generally have less cholesterol and saturated fat in their pattern of eating.

A vegetarian program isn't practical as a recommendation for the American public, so scientists attempted to recreate the vegetarian program while permitting some meat. They looked for the substances in the food that might explain the fall in blood pressure.

A nutritional program with more fruits and vegetables has more potassium. The level of potassium in the diet has definitely been shown to affect blood pressure. The higher the potassium, the lower the blood pressure. So this may be a partial explanation for the lowering, but it's not the entire story because feeding similar amounts of potassium doesn't lower the blood pressure to the same extent.

The other important nutrients found in vegetables and fruits are calcium and magnesium. However, studies haven't shown that these minerals lower blood pressure. Fat intake reduction and the increase in fiber may lower blood pressure, but their role in blood pressure control hasn't been determined either.

The people who designed DASH decided that it might be something in the mix of different nutrients that was responsible for the blood-pressure-lowering effect. They decided to try it on a large group of people with an emphasis on African Americans who have the highest rate of high blood pressure.

Proving the value of DASH

The study involved 459 people. They had to have a systolic blood pressure under 160 mm Hg and a diastolic blood pressure of 80 to 95 mm Hg. They were all older than 22, took no medications for high blood pressure, and had to stop taking any vitamins or food supplements. They couldn't drink more than 14 drinks of wine or other spirits per week. They couldn't have poorly controlled diabetes, high blood fats, or a body mass index greater than 35 (see Table 9-5). Two out of three participants were African Americans. The mean age was 44.

The average blood pressure of the group was 132/85 mm Hg with 29 percent having mild high blood pressure. They were mildly overweight with an average body mass index of 27. Twenty-seven percent were also smokers.

The participants followed the diets closely. They were given a three-week program of a usual American diet then randomly broken down into three groups. One group continued the usual American diet. The second group received a diet rich in fruits and vegetables while the third group was given DASH. All were followed for 8 weeks. They were given sufficient food so that they didn't lose weight and didn't have a decrease in salt intake.

After only 2 weeks, the usual diet group showed no change in blood pressure while the fruits and vegetables group reduced their blood pressures. But the greatest reduction in blood pressure was in the DASH group. This was sustained for the entire study, which lasted eight weeks.

The average reduction in blood pressure was 6/3 mm Hg, but the best results were among the people with the highest blood pressures, where it was 11/6 mm Hg.

Since the DASH study, other studies have accomplished the same excellent results using DASH, whether in an academic setting or in a primary care outpatient practice. Some of these studies have shown other beneficial effects of DASH.

DASH has lowered total blood cholesterol and low-density lipoprotein (LDL) or "bad" cholesterol. Blood levels of *homocysteine,* a substance associated with higher levels of coronary heart disease, have also been lowered.

Because most high blood pressure patients have mild Stage 1 high blood pressure (140 to 159 mm Hg for systolic blood pressure or 90 to 99 mm Hg for diastolic blood pressure, whichever is higher), and most of the illness and death occurs in that group, a lowering of blood pressure to the extent accomplished by DASH has the potential to have a significant impact on the health of Americans, especially those most at risk for the negative impact of high blood pressure.

A second study called DASH-Sodium, using various levels of sodium with the DASH program, showed that the lowest sodium level — 1,500 mg daily — lowered blood pressure even more.

Getting with the program

The DASH program is usually based on a 2,000-kilocalorie-a-day diet. If you need fewer kilocalories to maintain your weight, you should take the lower number of servings. If you need more kilocalories, take the higher number of servings.

If you find that following DASH is too difficult, don't hesitate to ask your doctor for a referral to a dietitian.

The 2,000 kilocalorie DASH eating plan has the following foods and servings:

- **7 to 8 servings of grains and grain products daily**

  A serving is 1 slice of bread, ½ bagel, ½ cup dry cereal, ½ cup cooked rice, pasta, or other cereal

- **4 to 5 servings of vegetables daily**

  A serving is 1 cup of raw leafy vegetables, ½ cup cooked vegetables, 6 ounces vegetable juice

- **4 to 5 servings of fruit daily**

  A serving is 6 ounces of fruit juice, 1 medium fruit, ½ cup dried fruit, ½ cup of fresh, frozen, or canned fruit

- **2 to 3 servings of low-fat or nonfat dairy products daily**

  A serving is 1 cup 1 percent milk, 1 cup low-fat yogurt, and 1.5 ounces nonfat cheese

- **2 or fewer servings of meats, poultry, or fish daily**

  A serving is 3 ounces of cooked lean meat, fish, or poultry

- **2½ servings of fats**

  A serving is 1 tsp oil, butter, margarine, mayonnaise, or 1 tbsp regular or 2 tbsp light salad dressing

- **4 to 5 servings of nuts, seeds, or legumes per week**

  A serving is ⅓ cup nuts, 2 tablespoons seeds, ½ cup cooked legumes, or 3 ounces tofu

✔ **5 servings of sweets per week including 1 tbsp sugar, 1 tbsp jelly or jam, ½ ounce jelly beans, or 8 ounces of lemonade**

Examples of good food choices in each group include

- ✔ **Grains and grain products:** Whole wheat breads, English muffins, pita bread, high-fiber cereals, and oatmeal
- ✔ **Vegetables:** Tomatoes, potatoes, carrots, peas, squash, broccoli, turnip greens, collards, kale, spinach, artichokes, green beans, and sweet potatoes
- ✔ **Fruits:** Apples, apricots, bananas, dates, grapes, oranges, orange juice, grapefruit, grapefruit juice, mangos, melons, peaches, pineapples, prunes, raisins, strawberries, and tangerines
- ✔ **Dairy products:** Skim or 1 percent milk, skim or low-fat buttermilk, nonfat or low-fat yogurt, part-skim mozzarella cheese and nonfat cheese
- ✔ **Meats, poultry, and fish:** Lean meats, poultry without skin, and no frying or sautéing
- ✔ **Nuts, seeds, and legumes:** Almonds, mixed nuts, peanuts, peanut butter, walnuts, sesame or sunflower seeds, kidney beans, pinto beans, navy beans, lentils, split peas, garbanzo beans, and tofu

To make up your daily nutrition, Table 9-2 shows a sample menu from which you can fill in the blanks.

Table 9-2	2,000 kilocalorie DASH menu		
Breakfast	*Lunch*	*Dinner*	*Snack*
2 grains	1 meat	1 meat	1 fruit
1 dairy	1 dairy	3 grains	1 grain
2 fruits	1 grain	2 vegetables	1 nuts
1 grain	1 fat	1 vegetable	
1 fat	1 vegetable	1½ fat servings	
	1 fruit	1 fruit	

Eat a snack once daily.

The menu can then be filled out as shown in Table 9-3 or you can have an entirely different day of meals as shown in Table 9-4.

Table 9-3	Example of a 2,000 kilocalorie DASH meal plan		
Breakfast	*Lunch*	*Dinner*	*Snack*
1 cup corn flakes	2 oz chicken	3 oz salmon	medium apple
1 cup 1% milk	½ oz cheddar	1 cup rice	1 slice wheat bread
1 banana	1 pita bread	1 cup squash	⅛ cup pecans
1 slice wheat toast	1 tsp margarine	1 cup spinach	
1 tbsp jam	1 cup raw carrots	1 tbsp light Italian dressing	
6 oz apple juice	1 orange	1½ oz low-fat Jack cheese	
1 tsp margarine			

Table 9-4	Another example of a 2,000 kilocalorie DASH meal plan		
Breakfast	*Lunch*	*Dinner*	*Snack*
1 cup prune juice	2 oz lean beef	3 oz trout	1 orange
1 cup oatmeal	1 tsp BBQ sauce	cup brown rice	1 oz dried fruit
slice whole wheat	roll	three-bean salad	2 tablespoons sunflower seeds
1 tsp margarine	1 cup boiled potatoes	low-fat dressing	
1 cup 1% milk	low-fat cheddar	1½ oz corn muffin	
1 banana	lettuce salad	1 tsp margarine	
	low-fat dressing	cup spinach	
	cup cranberry juice		

As you follow this diet you can make it easier for yourself in a variety of ways:

✔ Don't try to change all at once. Gradually reduce your meats and increase your fruits and vegetables.

✔ Make it easier to increase fruit and vegetable servings by having two at each meal and two for a snack.

✔ If you're lactose intolerant, take lactase pills with the dairy foods or buy lactose-free milk.

✔ Use the percent Daily Values on food labels to pick the foods that are lowest in saturated fats, total fats, cholesterol, and salt.

✔ Reduce your fats so that you're eating half as much and emphasize vegetable over animal fats.

✔ Avoid soda, alcohol, and other sugar-sweetened drinks.

✔ Use fruits as desserts.

✔ Make grains, such as pasta and rice or beans and vegetables, the center of the meal rather than meat, fish, or poultry.

Reducing salt as you DASH

Chapter 10 tells you all about salt and high blood pressure. The bottom line is the less salt in your diet, the lower your blood pressure. If you want to combine DASH with low salt, here are some suggestions:

✔ Products that you buy should say "Reduced sodium" or "No-salt added" on their labels.

✔ Use herbs, spices, a little wine, lemon, lime, or vinegar instead of salt to flavor your food.

✔ Leave the saltshaker in the kitchen, away from the table, to help you fight the urge to add more salt before eating.

✔ The more unprocessed foods you eat, the less salt you eat.

✔ Avoid high-salt condiments, such as soy sauce, teriyaki sauce, and MSG.

✔ Reduce your intake of salt-cured foods, foods in brine and mustard, horseradish, ketchup, and Worcestershire sauce.

✔ Reduce salt in recipes and replace it with other flavor enhancers.

✔ Eat fruit and vegetable snacks rather than salty snack foods.

✔ Be careful to avoid salty foods when eating out.

Reducing Your Weight Can Lower Blood Pressure

The fatter you are, the higher your blood pressure. More than 50 percent of the population is now overweight or obese as defined by the body mass index (BMI). (See Table 9-5 to look at the body mass index.) In this section, you can discover how to calculate your BMI. You can find out whether your weight falls within the range of acceptable weights for your height, and you'll find out how to calculate the number of kilocalories you need to lose weight if you are heavy or maintain a normal weight if not.

Weighing in

In order to use weight loss to lower your blood pressure, you need to know what your ideal weight should be. If you're already within the correct range of weights for your height, it's not likely that further weight loss can lower your blood pressure much more. If you're overweight or obese, weight loss to your ideal range significantly lowers your blood pressure.

Based on studies of many healthy men and women, your ideal weight range can be determined in the following manner:

✔ If you're a woman, give yourself 100 pounds for being 5 feet tall and add 5 pounds for every inch over 5 feet. For example, if you're 5 feet 3 inches, your appropriate weight is 115 pounds. The appropriate range is that weight plus or minus 10 percent. The appropriate range for a woman who is 5 feet 3 inches tall would be 104 to 126 pounds.

✔ If you're a man, give yourself 106 pounds for being 5 feet tall and 6 pounds more for every inch over 5 feet. A 5-foot-6-inch male should weigh about 142 pounds. The appropriate weight range is then 128 to 156 pounds.

You can also use your BMI to determine if you're under or overweight. The BMI is a number that takes into account your height to determine whether your weight is too high. This is only fair. A 5-foot-4-inch woman who weighs 150 pounds is overweight but a 5-foot-9-inch woman who weighs the same isn't overweight.

If you're good at math (or good with a calculator), you can determine your BMI for yourself. (In case you forget to carry the 1, I've done the work for you in Table 9-5.) Take your weight in pounds and multiply it by 705. Divide the result by your height in inches. Divide that result by your height in inches again. This is your body mass index in meters per kilogram squared. (Transferring pounds and inches into kilograms and meters is accomplished by the 705-fudge factor.)

REMEMBER

By definition, a BMI of 25 to 29.9 is an overweight BMI, and a BMI of 30 or greater is obese. A BMI of 20 to 25 is normal in weight.

So, for example, a 150-pound woman with a height of 5 feet and 4 inches or 64 inches is overweight with a BMI of 27.5. A 150-pound woman with a height of 5 feet and 9 inches or 69 inches has a normal BMI of 22.2.

If you prefer the easy way of determining your BMI, use Table 9-5. Find your height in inches or meters in the left hand column of Table 9-5. Move along that row until you reach your weight. Your BMI is found at the top of that column.

Table 9-5						Body Mass Index Chart								
	Body Mass Index (kg/ms²)													
	19	20	21	22	23	24	25	26	27	28	29	30	35	40
Height (inches/ meters)	*Body Weight (pounds)*													
58/1.47	91	96	100	105	110	115	119	124	129	134	138	143	167	191
59/1.50	94	99	104	109	114	119	124	128	133	138	143	148	173	198
60/1.52	97	102	107	112	118	123	128	133	138	143	148	153	179	204
61/1.55	100	106	111	116	122	127	132	137	143	148	153	158	185	211
62/1.57	104	109	115	120	126	131	136	142	147	153	158	164	191	218
63/1.60	107	113	118	124	130	135	141	146	152	158	163	169	197	225
64/1.63	110	116	122	128	134	140	145	151	157	163	169	174	204	232
65/1.65	114	120	126	132	138	144	150	156	162	168	174	180	210	240
66/1.68	118	124	130	136	142	148	155	161	167	173	179	186	216	247
67/1.70	121	127	134	140	146	153	159	166	172	178	185	191	223	255
68/1.73	125	131	138	144	151	158	164	171	177	184	190	197	230	262
69/1.75	128	135	142	149	155	162	169	176	182	189	196	203	236	270
70/1.78	132	139	146	153	160	167	174	181	188	195	202	207	243	278
71/1.80	136	143	150	157	165	172	179	186	193	200	208	215	250	286
72/1.83	140	147	154	162	169	177	184	191	199	206	213	221	258	294
73/1.85	144	151	159	166	174	182	189	197	204	212	219	227	265	302
74/1.8836p	148	155	163	171	179	186	194	202	210	218	225	233	272	311
75/1.90	152	160	168	176	184	192	200	208	216	224	232	240	279	319
76/1.93	156	164	172	180	189	197	205	213	221	230	238	246	287	328

Determining your daily caloric needs

Caloric needs are different for different ages, sexes, and levels of activity. For example, if a woman is pregnant or breast-feeding, she obviously needs more kilocalories. If a person is trying to lose weight, then reducing the total kilocalories per day can accomplish this. After you know your appropriate weight for your height, you can determine the number of kilocalories that you require each day to maintain that weight as well as the reduction in kilocalories that can result in weight loss. This may best be done with a dietitian to make sure you're getting the right nutrients while staying within your daily caloric limits.

A pound of fat contains 3,500 kilocalories. To lose a pound of fat, therefore, you must eat 3,500 kilocalories less than you need. You can do this by a daily reduction of 500 kilocalories for seven days or by doing 200 kilocalories of exercise a day and reducing the diet by only 300 kilocalories daily. For most people, a combination of diet and exercise seems to work much better than diet alone.

You don't have to lose weight all the way down to your appropriate range to benefit from weight loss. A loss of 5 to 10 percent of your current weight brings important benefits in terms of blood pressure, blood fats, and blood glucose if diabetes is present.

Imagine, for example, a 5-foot-3-inch woman who weighs 150 pounds. Her appropriate weight is 115 pounds within a range of 104 to 126 pounds.

If this woman weighed 115 pounds, she would require 115×10 or 1,150 kilocalories plus more depending on her level of exercise. If she is sedentary, she's entitled to 10 percent more kilocalories for a total of about 1,265 kilocalories daily. If she is moderately active, she gets 20 percent more for a total of 1,380 kilocalories daily. A very active woman may need 40 percent or more extra kilocalories to cover her exercise needs. This would take her up to 1,610 kilocalories. By reducing her daily intake to 1,400 while doing 300 kilocalories of exercise daily, she will lose a pound of fat a week.

After you have the total kilocalories, you can go back to the DASH program and subtract or add servings appropriately. If you want to try to figure out the DASH program at a lower caloric range without the assistance of a dietitian, here's some help. Table 9-6 shows the breakdown of servings for a 2,000, 1,800, and 1,500 kilocalorie DASH program.

Table 9-6	Servings Comparison for 2,000, 1,8 and 1,500 kilocalorie DASH		
Food Group	**2,000 kilocalorie servings**	**1,800 kilocalorie servings**	**1,500 kilocalorie servings**
Grains	8	8	5.5
Vegetables	4	4	4
Fruits	5	4	4
Dairy foods	3	3	3
Meats and fish	2	1¾	1¾
Fats and oils	2½	2½	1½
Nuts and seeds	1	1	¾
Sweets	5 per week		

Trying Other Diets

Sometimes you need a boost to get you going in the right direction towards weight loss and the resulting reduction in blood pressure. I don't insist that my patients follow a balanced nutrition plan all the time as long as I'm certain that they're generally getting the good nutrition they need. A special plan may be what you need to get you started, and then you can continue on a healthy, balanced program, such as DASH. For example, one of my patients eats nothing but rice and water one week a month, eating balanced meals the rest of the time. He has lost a significant amount of weight, come off all blood pressure medication, and has a blood pressure anyone would envy. He looks and feels great.

Weight loss is difficult for many reasons. In my experience, most patients do well initially but tend to return to old habits. Still, losing weight and keeping it off is definitely possible. At one time, it was calculated that only one out of twenty people who lost weight would keep it off. Now the figure is closer to one in five.

Successfully losing weight and maintaining it also requires a willingness to exercise. Chapter 12 is all about exercise both for health and for weight loss. If, for some reason, you can't move your legs to exercise, you can get a satisfactory workout using your upper body. When people who are successful at weight loss maintenance are questioned, most of them describe exercise as a key part of their success.

The diets I describe aren't balanced diets and shouldn't be your nutritional plan for more than several weeks to get you going. They're generally associated with regaining the weight if they become your primary program. They're usually boring, repetitious, and have little to do with the pleasure of eating.

- **Very-low-kilocalorie diets:** These diets provide 400 to 800 kilocalories a day of protein and carbohydrate with supplemental vitamins and minerals. They're safe when supervised by a physician and used when you need rapid weight loss, such as in the case of a heart condition. They result in rapid initial weight loss with a fall in the need for medication for high blood pressure. In fact, if you continue your medication, you may suffer dizziness.

- **Animal-protein diets** (such as the Atkins diet): Food is limited to animal protein in an effort to maintain body protein, along with vitamins and minerals. Patients often complain of hair loss. Weight is rapidly regained when the diet is discontinued. This isn't a balanced diet.

- **Fasts:** A fast means giving up all food for a period of time and taking only water and vitamins and minerals. A fast is such a drastic change from normal eating habits that most patients do not remain on the fast for very long and weight is regained.

Using Outside Help

The dietitian can be a tremendous source of information on all aspects of nutrition. He can help you determine your correct weight and how many kilocalories per day are needed to reach that weight. Other programs have also proved to be valuable for some people. Many of these programs provide all the food that you care to eat, making it exceedingly easy to follow them (although they can also be exceedingly expensive). These programs emphasize gradual weight loss and a connection to more normal eating habits, both of which seem to be a more successful way to lose weight.

- **Jenny Craig:** This organization provides the food that you eat, which you must pay for. It offers information on food behavior modification.

- **Weight Watchers:** This organization emphasizes slow weight loss, exercise, and behavior modification. It charges for weekly attendance at its meetings, which you can find all over the world. It doesn't require that you purchase any products. Foods are available for purchase. It has developed a point program that allows you to eat what you want so long as the total is within the points that you're allowed each day. After you reach your goal weight, you can belong for free as long as you stay at that weight or near it. Weight Watchers is very motivating.

Characteristics of successful losers

What is it about the people who've lost weight and kept it off that's different from you or me, or perhaps just me? The National Weight Loss Registry set out to find out how they do it. They have surveyed more than 3,000 people who've lost at least 30 pounds and have kept it off for at least one year.

The people had a starting BMI of 36 and currently had a BMI of 25 on average. They had lost an average of 71 pounds. Here are some of their characteristics:

- 74 percent had one or both overweight parents.
- 20 percent were overweight by age 18.
- They had recycled (gained and lost) an average of 271 pounds over their lifetime.
- Most had lost weight in the usual ways, by restricting foods, portion control, counting kilocalories and limiting fats.
- Their average kilocalorie intake was 1,400 kilocalories per day.
- Their average weekly kilocalorie expenditure from exercise was 2,800 kilocalories.
- 55 percent used a program such as Weight Watchers, Overeaters Anonymous, or a dietitian.
- 45 percent lost weight on their own.
- 77 percent reported a medical or emotional trigger causing them to finally lose weight successfully.

If you study these characteristics, you find that these people aren't doing strange things to lose weight. They're using ordinary nutritional plans that are usually balanced along with exercise and sometimes outside help.

Chapter 10

Salt and High Blood Pressure

· ·

In This Chapter

▶ Tracing salt in human history

▶ Finding out how salt raises your blood pressure

▶ Studying the effect of salt consumption and salt sensitivity

▶ Eating salt to live instead of living to eat salt

· ·

The Salt Institute, a nonprofit association of salt producers founded in 1914, would have you believe that eating salt doesn't raise your blood pressure, and that if it does, proof that the result is harmful to your health doesn't exist. Don't believe them! With rare exceptions, every expert in the field of high blood pressure recommends reducing salt consumption to lower high blood pressure.

The United States is by far the world's largest producer of salt. We make about 45 million metric tons annually compared with the next country, China, which makes 28 million metric tons followed by Germany at 16 million, India at 14 million, Canada at 12 million, and Australia at 10 million. These six countries account for 125 million of the 209 million metric tons produced each year in the world. Only 6 percent of that salt is used for human consumption. The countries that produce the most tend to consume the most per person — a situation that helps to explain the high prevalence of high blood pressure in those countries.

In this chapter, you find out that your salt intake can elevate your blood pressure and that research has provided overwhelming evidence to this effect. Reading this chapter, you also discover how a sensitivity to salt can increase your blood pressure, how to decrease the amount of salt in your food, what foods are low in salt and what foods are high in salt, and what's in a low-salt diet. You *can* eat without salting down your plate. Hopefully, by the end of the chapter, you'll put your saltshaker away, never to be seen again, orat least reduce your salt intake, so that it doesn't do you any harm.

Making the Connection between Salt and High Blood Pressure

Salt, which is made up of 40 percent sodium and 60 percent chloride, is critical to your life. You can't live without it. Sodium helps to maintain your blood's water content, serves to balance the acids and bases in your blood, and is necessary for the movement of electrical charges in the nerves that move our muscles.

It's generally believed that the inability of your kidney to excrete salt is responsible for salt-induced high blood pressure. By increasing blood pressure, more salt is filtered by the kidney, enters the urine, and the body compensates for its inability to excrete salt. This increased blood pressure helps to eliminate more salt, but it also puts a strain on your arteries and sets the downward spiral of blood-pressure damage in motion — a vicious cycle.

The recommendation for salt in the Dietary Guidelines for Americans from the U.S. Department of Health and Human Services as well as the American Heart Association is 2,400 milligrams (mg) daily for adults. This is the amount in 1 teaspoon of salt (2,300 mg to be exact). The average American consumes 5,000 mg of salt daily — twice the necessary amount. Normal salt balance can be maintained with 500 mg daily (or a little more than one-fourth teaspoon of salt), so Americans are eating ten times as much as they really need. Canada, Australia, the United Kingdom, and Portugal all have about the same recommendation of 2,400 mg of salt. Some countries, such as Germany (4,000 mg), the Netherlands (3,600 mg) and Belgium (3,500 mg), are more liberal and at least one country, Sweden (800 mg), is more restrictive than the United States.

"Where is all this salt coming from?" you may ask. Many foods are a natural source of salt (such as meat and fish) while others contain salt added during processing (prepared soup and crackers, for example). For more information on the amount of salt in the foods you eat, see the "Lowering Your Salt Intake" section, later in this chapter.

Determining If You're Salt Sensitive

Salt was first shown to raise blood pressure in experiments with rats in the *Journal of the American Dietetic Association* (February 1957). Those rats that were fed the most salt had the highest blood pressure at the end of nine months. Not all rats show this increase in blood pressure, however. Some are sensitive to salt and some aren't. It was shown that the sensitivity was hereditary, that is, passed down through the genes.

Salt sensitivity in humans is similar. When children of parents with high blood pressure eat salt in large quantities, they can't get rid of it through their urine as rapidly as children of parents who don't have high blood pressure. Similarly, when children of parents with high blood pressure are given salt, their blood pressure is higher if both parents have high blood pressure than if only one parent has high blood pressure. When children of parents without high blood pressure are given salt in large quantities, their blood pressure isn't elevated at all. These findings are published in the *Journal of Hypertension* (April 1986).

About half the U.S. population (and, where studied, the populations in other industrialized countries) is salt sensitive. This has caused plenty of confusion in experiments meant to show the effects of salt on human beings. The most salt sensitive people are African Americans, people over age 65, and those who have diabetes.

You should reduce your salt intake whether you're salt sensitive or not. If you are, it will help to reduce your blood pressure. If not, it will reduce the extra water that's retained as a result of the increased salt intake.

At first glance, the evidence for the connection between excess salt and high blood pressure would seem overwhelming. However, a few studies seem to show that salt isn't dangerous to your health. In one particular study reported in *Hypertension* (June 1995), Alderman wrote that heart attacks increased among the group of men who had the lowest salt intake. This study has a number of problems associated with it. The most serious problem was that the results were based on a test of a single specimen for the amount of salt that a person consumed although the study went on for four years after that test.

Proving the Salt-Blood Pressure Connection

An experiment that involved the consumption of an overabundance of salt would be hard to do on human beings because their salt intake is so high to begin with, and it would take an unpalatable amount of additional salt to raise the body's salt level significantly.

Although reducing your salt intake hasn't been proven to lower your blood pressure, studies have shown that eating less salt, in most cases, leads to lower blood pressure and fewer instances of heart attack and brain attack. For example, the blood pressure measurements of individuals with a great craving for salt have been extremely high during periods when they ate an abundance of salt. Then the same individuals stopped eating salt; blood pressures dropped significantly when the salt was reduced. Studies of people with high blood pressure who undergo periods of salt reduction are more easily done. In the early twentieth-century, the first experiments on the salt-blood pressure connection showed that blood pressure fell as salt was reduced. These studies can be found in the *Archives of General Medicine* (February 1904).

A low-salt diet lowered blood pressure in up to half of patients with high blood pressure. In the rest of the patients, changes may have occurred that were irreversible, such that the blood pressure would no longer respond to salt deprivation alone or some may not have been salt sensitive.

In the *American Journal of Medicine* (March 1948), a study established without a doubt that salt restriction lowers blood pressure. Shortly thereafter, however, the first *diuretics* (blood pressure drugs that increase salt and water excretion; see Chapter 13) were marketed and the salt restriction as a means of lowering blood pressure fell out of favor. As side effects from the drugs became a problem, however, salt restriction became more popular again.

In 1988, the Intersalt Study, a huge study of over 10,000 people from many nations, showed that salt intake is directly related to the rise of both systolic and diastolic blood pressures with age. The researchers believe that a reduction of 1 teaspoon of salt intake daily from age 25 to 55 can reduce the blood pressure by 9 mm Hg. People who lived where the salt intake was lowest had no increase in blood pressure with age.

Salt through human history

Human beings who lived away from the seashores several thousand years ago didn't eat much salt because most salt comes from the sea. They existed on no more than 200 to 400 milligrams (or less than half a teaspoon) of salt each day. The human body generally conserves salt. When an athlete sweats, he puts out sweat with less and less salt as exercise continues. Meanwhile, the kidneys are returning all the filtered salt back to the body.

When the discovery was made that adding salt preserved and extended the life of some foods, salt became much more valuable. At the same time, the salty taste of food became the norm and unsalted food was considered bland. Salt became such a sought-after commodity that governments began to put a tax on salt transactions to gain revenue. The salt tax was a major reason for the French Revolution.

As methods of producing salt improved, it became cheap. Salt consumption rose enormously. By the nineteenth century, people consumed as much as 20 grams (or 4 teaspoons) of salt daily. Luckily, with refrigeration, adding salt as a preservative to food began to decline.

Current professional opinion maintains that sodium alone doesn't raise blood pressure. Rather, the combination of sodium and chloride is what raises blood pressure. Studies at the University of California in San Francisco by Dr. R. Curtis Morris and his associates have shown that some people are sensitive to both sodium and chloride, but some are sensitive to chloride even when it's not combined with sodium. Morris and his associates found, for example, that potassium chloride, often given to replace the sodium in sodium chloride, which is salt, can raise blood pressure in rats that are genetically prone to high blood pressure just as much as sodium chloride. Whether this is applicable to human beings is uncertain at the present time. Ten years ago, Morris and his associates showed that sodium bicarbonate (baking soda) does not raise blood pressure in salt-sensitive people. They recommend that potassium bicarbonate or potassium citrate replace sodium chloride rather than potassium chloride.

A study of people with high blood pressure in Germany found in *Hypertension* (October 1990) offers evidence that chloride plays a part in high blood pressure. A group of patients with high blood pressure were given potassium chloride or potassium citrate. Those who received potassium citrate lowered their blood pressure significantly, but those who received potassium chloride in place of sodium chloride did not. The potassium in fruits and vegetables is not potassium chloride. This may help to explain the positive effects of fruits and vegetables on high blood pressure.

Lowering Your Salt Intake

Surprisingly, you're responsible for only 15 percent of the salt in your diet. Food has about 10 percent of your salt already naturally in it. The food industry is responsible for adding 75 percent of the salt that you consume each day to the prepared foods that you buy. For example, the following additives contain plenty of salt:

- **Color Developer:** Promotes the development of color in meats and sauerkraut.
- **Fermentation Controller:** In cheeses, sauerkraut, and baked goods.
- **Binder:** To keep meat together as it cooks.
- **Texture Aid:** Allows dough to expand and not tear.

For these and other reasons, salt is part of food processing. It may not be for taste.

The only way that you can successfully reduce the salt in your diet is by switching from processed foods to fresh foods or selecting low-salt processed foods.

Buying low-salt foods

The Food and Drug Administration has definite guidelines as to the terms a food company can use when describing the salt in the food on the label. Keep these terms in mind and make a point of buying low-salt foods on your next trip to the grocery store.

- **Sodium free** means less than 5 mg sodium in a portion.

- **Very low sodium** means less than 35 mg sodium in a portion.

- **Low sodium** means less than 140 mg sodium in a portion.

- **Reduced sodium** food contains 25 percent less sodium than the original food item.

- **Light in sodium** food has 50 percent less sodium than the original food item.

- **Unsalted, No salt added,** or **Without added salt** means absolutely no salt has been added to a food that's normally processed with salt.

Combining a low-salt diet with DASH

Chapter 9 explained the DASH nutritional program in detail. Combine DASH with a low-salt diet to get the maximum blood pressure-lowering effect. Some recommendations for the various food groups in DASH are as follows:

- **Grain group:** Check the salt content of any prepared grain foods, and keep the sodium less than 180 mg in each serving. Avoid any salted grain foods, such as salted popcorn.

- **Fruit group:** Avoid dried fruits with salt.

- **Vegetable group:** Eat fresh vegetables, and read the label on prepared vegetables.

- **Meat group:** Eat fresh meats, fish, and poultry; avoid salt-cured products.

- **Dairy group:** Read the label, and avoid products with more than 180 mg of sodium per serving.

- **Fat group:** Avoid high-salt salad dressings and salted butter.

- **Nuts and seeds:** Avoid salted varieties.

- **Sweets:** Check the box, and stay away from prepared mixes that contain more than 180 mg of sodium per serving.

Take time to read the Nutrition Facts label on food items. Avoid items that contain more than 180 milligrams of sodium.

Avoiding high-salt foods

Table 10-1 shows you the processed foods that are particularly high in salt. Avoid eating these foods as much as possible. Fortunately, after many years of urging and recommendations from health organizations, manufacturers have begun to lower the salt in foods, so you may find several of these foods in a low-salt form. Check the food label.

Table 10-1	Prepared High-Salt Foods	
Anchovies	Condiments	Pickles
Bacon	Cooking sauces	Salad dressings
Bouillon cubes	Cottage cheese	Salsa
Canned soups	Croutons	Sausage
Canned tuna	Gravy	Sea salt
Canned vegetables	Ham	Soy sauce
Cheese	Hot dogs	Spaghetti sauce
Cold cuts	Olives	Tomato or vegetable juice

Going on a low-salt diet

Besides avoiding high-salt foods, you can make a few other changes to lower your salt intake:

- Cook with herbs, spices, fruit juices, and vinegars for flavor rather than salt.
- Eat fresh vegetables.
- Keep the saltshaker in the kitchen cupboard rather than at the table, where it's so easy to use.
- Use less salt than the recipe calls for.

✔ Select low-salt canned foods or rinse your food with water.

✔ Select low-salt frozen dinners.

✔ Use high-salt condiments, such as ketchup and mustard, sparingly.

✔ Snack on fresh fruits rather than salted crackers or chips.

✔ When eating out, ask that your food be prepared with only a little salt. Request your salad dressing "on the side" of the salad, so you can control the amount that goes on it.

Be careful of salt substitutes. Some contain sodium. Check the label. You could end up eating so much of the substitute in an attempt to get that salty taste that your total sodium intake is just as high as using salt.

Chapter 11

Avoiding Poison: Tobacco, Alcohol, and Caffeine

Suppose I told you that if you're older than 45 years of age, you could do all of the following:

- ✔ Improve your work performance, your sex life, and the health of you and your baby if pregnant

- ✔ Increase your social activities and the possibility of living longer

- ✔ Reduce the possibility of getting a driving ticket, of contracting a sexually-transmitted disease, and of suicide or homicide

- ✔ Lower your blood pressure

Would you make a little sacrifice? Of course, you would. All that you need to do is quit smoking (or chewing smokeless tobacco), stop drinking excessively, and stop drinking coffee. You're probably thinking that's easy for me to say but much harder for you to do. Lucky for you, I give you every available tool to make this lifestyle improvement as easy as possible. Nothing you could ever do for your health can make a greater difference than cutting out tobacco, alcohol, and caffeine.

In this chapter, I take up each one of these dangerous habits individually and discuss how they affect your blood pressure. I also discuss how eliminating these poisons from your life can help lower your blood pressure and make your mind and body healthier in the process.

Keep in mind that tobacco, alcohol, and caffeine most often go together. The person who smokes more often than not is the person who drinks too much alcohol and too much caffeine. Tobacco, alcohol, and caffeine represent a triple threat to your health. But within that triple threat may also be triple salvation. Reducing or eliminating one of these three poisons often leads to a reduction or elimination of one or both of the others. The tendency to have that cigarette with your scotch or your coffee is eliminated if you don't drink the scotch or the coffee.

Playing with Fire

When you play with fire, you get burned. When you smoke, you run the risk of getting burned inside and out. Whether tobacco is smoked or chewed or taken in by any other means, the nicotine in the tobacco raises the blood pressure. The more you smoke, the higher the nicotine level is in your blood, and the higher your blood pressure. This accounts to a large extent for the great increase in brain attacks (see Chapter 7), heart attacks and pain in the legs due to poor circulation in smokers, sometimes leading to amputation.

Nicotine raises your blood pressure by constricting your blood vessels. This occurs because the oxygen in your blood decreases and because nicotine directly stimulates the production of a hormone, *epinephrine* (also known as adrenaline), in the adrenal gland. Epinephrine raises blood pressure. After tobacco use raises blood pressure, you're at risk of all the medical consequences of high blood pressure (described in Part II), not to mention diseases associated with smoking, such as mouth and lung cancer.

Numerous studies have shown that smoking or chewing tobacco raises blood pressure and that when you stop using tobacco products, your blood pressure falls. The latest such study in the *Journal of Hypertension* (February 2002) comes from France. Out of 12,417 men who were current smokers, previous smokers, and never smokers, current smokers had the highest prevalence of high blood pressure. Previous smokers had a lower prevalence with the highest rate of high blood pressure in those who had recently stopped and had smoked for the longest time. Those who had never started smoking had the lowest prevalence of high blood pressure. Do you need more evidence than that?

Cigarettes (and smokeless tobacco like chewing tobacco) deserve their own book, but I give you enough evidence of the dangers of tobacco and enough helpful advice to quit using tobacco that you would have to be a real dummy not to stop immediately, if not sooner. Drugs that have caused a small fraction of the illness and death that tobacco can be blamed for have been taken off the market. So why are cigarettes still sold legally and advertised in many of our most prestigious magazines? The answer to that question lies squarely at the feet of government and the millions of dollars spent on cigarettes that are turned around and used to influence that government. Some day you'll look back on these times and ask yourself, "Could I really have been that stupid?"

Examining the extent of the problem

Fifty million Americans smoked in 1996 — about the same number of people who have high blood pressure — although many with high blood pressure do not smoke, and some who smoke do not have high blood pressure. The problem is even greater in other countries. One third of the population of the world older than age 15 smokes, a total of 1.1 billion people. In many other countries, more than half the adult population smokes.

The overall rate of smoking in America has declined since 1993 from 25 percent to 22.3 percent in 2001 according to the U.S. smoking statistics of the National Institutes of Health. The federal government has set a goal of 12 percent by 2010. This won't be achieved if the current rate of fall in smoking continues. The decline in other countries has been even less.

In terms of the age of smokers, about 18 percent of youths age 12 to 17 years smoke, 38 percent of young adults age 18 to 25 years smoke, 27 percent of people age 26 to 44 years of age, and only 10 percent of adults aged 65+ continue to smoke. Most tobacco users begin before the age of 18 despite the continued "efforts" of the tobacco companies to avoid attracting that age group.

Native Americans lead among the various ethnic groups in percent of smokers at a rate of 41 percent while Caucasians and African Americans have the same rate of about 30 percent. About 25 percent of Hispanics are smokers while only 14 percent of Asians and Pacific Islanders are smokers.

People can stop smoking. The evidence is that 46 million former smokers were in the U.S. in 1999.

The direct costs of smoking, such as health insurance costs, use of medical care and expenses due to medical care amount to more than 50 billion dollars per year. The indirect costs, such as loss of work due to smoking-related illness and loss in productivity from deaths due to smoking, add another 80 billion or so dollars. Many experts suggest that a much higher tax on cigarettes should meet these costs in part. This would not only help to pay for the self-inflicted diseases of smokers but discourage the purchase of cigarettes in the first place. The current gradual decline in smoking among the population is the result of the last time that cigarette taxes were raised.

One of the earliest positive consequences of smoking cessation is a fall in blood pressure. However blood pressure is lowered, the medical consequences due to high blood pressure (discussed in Part II) become less likely.

Putting one foot in the grave

Blood pressure elevation is just one of smoking's many consequences. Other smoking-related complications are as follows.

- Lung cancer is 20 times more likely among smokers than nonsmokers.
- Cancers of the mouth and throat as well as the bladder are more likely among smokers. The connection isn't as clear, but smoking is also likely to increase the possibility of cancers of the liver, large intestine, pancreas, kidney, and the cervix in women.
- Coronary heart disease is much more common among smokers, whether they have increased blood pressure or not.
- Brain attacks (see Chapter 7) are more common among smokers — again, regardless of elevated blood pressure.
- Bleeding from rupture of the large blood vessel in the abdomen is more common.
- Chronic lung disease is most often the result of smoking.
- Lung growth rate is reduced among adolescents who smoke.
- Women who smoke have trouble conceiving a baby, and if they do, they're more likely to miscarry. Women who smoke also tend to start menopause at a younger age.
- Smoking reduces bone density and increases the risk of fractures in older women especially.
- A correlation exists between smoking and depression.

Do you need more reasons to stop smoking? Just keep this in mind: If you smoke, you're not utterly cool; you're an utter fool.

Dealing with secondhand smoke

Secondhand smoke, also called *environmental tobacco smoke,* is smoke that you inhale from someone else's cigarette. Secondhand smoke can be just as deadly as smoke from the other end of the cigarette and perhaps more so. The smoke is mostly unfiltered from the burning end of the cigarette, called *sidestream smoke.*

It's even more dangerous than mainstream smoke (from the nonburning end) because it contains more of the poisons. It causes 3,000 deaths annually due to lung cancer in nonsmokers. It's also been shown to cause 55,000 deaths annually in nonsmokers due to heart and blood vessel disease.

Nicotine is one of the many toxins that enter the air in secondhand smoke, doing its best to raise your blood pressure without your help. Don't become a victim of secondhand smoke.

- ✔ Allow no one to smoke in your home or car.
- ✔ Never smoke with children around.
- ✔ Improve ventilation if exposure to smoke can't be avoided.
- ✔ Insist that offices and bars be completely smoke-free.

Regarding smokeless tobacco

Smokeless tobacco is tobacco that you chew or put into your nostrils. Types of smokeless tobacco include snuff, which is placed between the cheek and the gum in the United States and is sniffed into the nose in Europe, and chewing tobacco, which is a wad of tobacco that is placed inside the cheek and chewed on to extract the juices. In the process of using either one, a great deal of saliva is produced forcing the user to spit frequently. Not a pretty picture.

Smokeless tobacco provides at least twice as much nicotine as a cigarette. Eight to ten chews a day is equivalent to 40 cigarettes a day in nicotine content. Therefore, using smokeless tobacco damages the heart and blood vessels over the long term, and the effect on the blood pressure is that much greater and of a longer duration. In addition, smokeless tobacco is filled with agents that cause cancer.

Smokeless tobacco won't help you quit smoking. Actually, smokeless tobacco is just as addictive as cigarettes if not more. So don't think that using smokeless tobacco instead of cigarettes can get rid of your nicotine cravings. Instead, smokeless tobacco discolors your teeth, sours your breath, and creates cancer in your throat, voice box, and esophagus.

Everything to gain and nothing to lose

Why should you give up something that you find pleasurable and that may even make it easier to keep those extra pounds off? As far as the pounds, you can get rid of those with more exercise and fewer kilocalories. As for the pleasure, the short and long-term health consequences when you quit are as follows:

- The healing starts within 12 hours as the carbon monoxide levels in your body fall and your heart and lungs begin to function more normally with a resultant fall in your blood pressure and your heart rate.

- Your taste buds and your sense of smell return in a few days

- Your face wrinkles far less as you age.

- If you're attempting to get pregnant, achieving pregnancy is easier; and after you're pregnant, the pregnancy proceeds in a healthier manner.

- Your smoker's cough diminishes after a few days, though it may last for a while as your rejuvenated lungs begin to mobilize and expel the gunk accumulated over years of smoking.

- The stench of stale smoke and the mess of cigarette butts will be gone along with the expense of smoking and the time wasted buying cigarettes and finding a place to smoke away from others.

- Your risk of early death is the same as that of a nonsmoker after 10 to 15 years of no cigarettes, depending on how long you smoked before stopping.

- After five years, the risk of cancer of the mouth and throat along with bladder cancer and cancer of the cervix in women is significantly diminished.

- After ten years, you have half the chance of developing lung cancer than if you continued to smoke.

Obviously, the healthy consequences of quitting tobacco should be reason enough for you to stop, but other reasons may help sway you just as much:

- A loved one may tell you that the cigarettes go or you go. After all, kissing a smoker is like licking an ashtray.

- The money saved from not smoking may provide a down payment for a new car, a new computer, or just allow you to keep eating.

- You freeze standing outside while getting your nicotine fix several times a day.

- The time saved not having to go to the store or stand outside can be used to exercise or do some other healthy activity.

- You're getting as disgusted as I am with the cigarette butts that litter city streets.

- Last but not least, the time that you add onto your life can't be totaled up in terms of just days but productive, healthy days — days that you otherwise may have spent gasping for breath with an oxygen tube in your nose, too short of breath to walk over to your grandchild and hug her.

Kicking the habit

The last few years have seen a smoking-cessation-treatment revolution. Nicotine gum followed what began as psychotherapy. Then came nicotine patches, and now, drugs that don't contain nicotine take away the craving for nicotine. In this section, you can find something that appeals to you. I know that you want to quit smoking because more than 70 percent of adults have expressed a desire to stop smoking. Now's your chance!

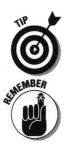

No one way works for all people. Try each one. If it doesn't work for you, try another technique. Something will click eventually.

You benefit from stopping smoking no matter what your age or physical condition.

Keys to quitting

You must take five steps to ensure that you quit and don't relapse or try again to quit if you do relapse. Follow these steps and your success is far more likely:

1. **Prepare yourself.**

   Set a quit date and make it special. After all, your body is being reborn. Your birth date would do nicely. It will be a day of celebration for the rest of your life.

   Make a list of reasons to quit. Improve your fitness, which makes any significant change easier to manage. Avoid drinks with caffeine to help you to sleep after you quit smoking. Satisfy your hunger with low-calorie beverages or snacks. Relax yourself by exercising, taking a bath, or meditation. Treat any cough with cough drops or hard candy.

2. **Benefit from the support of friends and loved ones.**

   Let everyone know you're quitting and ask for help, especially by not smoking in your presence. Even better, ask them to stop with you. Use individual or group counseling to support you. This may mean talking to someone as many as several times a day as you're trying to quit. Check with your doctor or other healthcare provider for ideas that she may have to help you.

3. **Use new skills to handle problems that arise.**

   Find distractions that substitute for the urge to smoke. Stop activities that you combine with smoking, such as drinking alcohol or coffee, the morning break, or whatever you know to be a smoking trigger. Change your routine to emphasize the lifestyle change. Find an enjoyable substitute for smoking. Switch to a brand that you don't like that's low nicotine before you stop. Smoke only half the cigarette. Limit yourself to an increasingly smaller fixed number of cigarettes daily. After you get down to seven or less, set a quit date. Drink plenty of noncaloric fluids, such as water.

4. **Make use of the medications that have proven to be effective in helping a person quit.**

Ask your doctor about nicotine replacement therapy and smoking cessation aids.

5. **Prepare for relapses.**

Everyone who has successfully quit smoking has probably done it on the second, third, or fourth try. Giving yourself another chance to succeed if things go wrong temporarily is essential. If you relapse, it usually occurs within the first three months. Meanwhile, you can avoid the situations where relapse is most likely:

- Try not to drink alcohol, which can lessen your control.

- Stay away from smokers. You don't even want a whiff of smoke.

- Don't return to smoking just because you gain weight. You can lose it sooner or later.

- Don't treat your nervousness, depression, or anxiety with a cigarette.

Should you relapse, begin the process of quitting again as soon as possible. The less you smoke, the easier it will be to quit again. Try to recognize the situations that blocked your success and avoid them the next time around.

Effective methods of quitting

Two effective methods for quitting smoking are nicotine replacement therapy and smoking cessation aids. Some methods can be bought over the counter while others require a prescription from your doctor. The details of each method are provided as follows:

- **Nicotine-replacement therapy:** The point of nicotine replacement therapy is to deliver small doses of nicotine to avoid withdrawal from tobacco. If you have high blood pressure associated with nicotine intake, you want to use nicotine replacement therapy as short a time as possible because nicotine in this form raises your blood pressure. You have four ways of doing this:

  - **Nicotine gum,** available over-the-counter, is sold in 2 mg and 4 mg strengths. By chewing it, nicotine is released and absorbed by the membranes in the mouth. By reducing the number of pieces each day, a day is reached when none are needed.

- **Nicotine patches,** available both by prescription and over-the-counter, release nicotine gradually through the skin. They come in 15 mg strength or in varying doses that decline as withdrawal from tobacco continues. People with allergies to adhesives will have trouble with this. Combining the gum and the patches may work better than either alone, but be sure to get your doctor's approval before using both treatments together.

- **Nicotine nasal spray** is available by prescription only. It is inhaled whenever there is an urge to smoke. It is difficult to use when there is a sinus condition.

- **Nicotine inhalers,** available by prescription, deliver nicotine in a vapor into the mouth where the membranes absorb it. It may irritate the mouth and throat.

✔ **Smoking-cessation aids:** Bupropion SR, tradename Zyban, acts to disrupt the addictive power of nicotine. At a dose of 300 mg, given as 150 mg twice daily, available by prescription, it has proved its effectiveness in large studies of smokers.

A combination of bupropion and a nicotine-replacement aid accomplished a much higher rate of quitting than either one did alone.

Tapping into resources

With the availability of the World Wide Web, you have many resources to help you quit smoking at the peck of a key on your computer keyboard. If you're computer-challenged, you can access these resources by mail or telephone. Here are the best of the lot:

✔ The National Institutes of Health contains the **National Cancer Institute** (NCI). The NCI does research on quitting smoking, promotes programs to decrease the impact of smoking on health, and publishes materials on the Internet and in hard copy with tips on quitting and avoiding secondhand smoke. The NCI supports the Cancer Information Service from which these materials are available at 1-800-4-Cancer. The Web address is http://cis.nci.nih.gov.

✔ **The National Institute on Drug Abuse** (NIDA) is another part of the National Institutes of Health. It supports research on cigarettes and other sources of nicotine as an addictive drug. Fact sheets are available concerning drug abuse and addition at 1-888-NIH-NIDA. The Web address is www.health.org.

✔ **The Office on Smoking and Health National Center for Chronic Disease Prevention** has a database of smoking and health-related materials at 1-800-232-1311 or on the Web at www.cdc.gov/tobacco.

 ✔ **The Agency for Healthcare Research and Quality** has smoking cessation guidelines and other materials for both physicians and the public at 1-800-358-9295 or on the Web at `www.ahcpr.gov`.

 ✔ **The American Cancer Society** has many pamphlets and Web pages on quitting smoking as well as a bibliography of books and tapes on quitting at 1-800-227-2345 or `www.cancer.org`.

 ✔ **The American Lung Association** has both information and clinics to help you stop smoking at 1-800-586-4872 or `www.lungusa.org`.

 ✔ **The American Heart Association** provides information on smoking-cessation programs in schools, workplaces, and healthcare sites. To obtain, call 1-800-242-8721 or visit the Internet at `www.americanheart.org`.

 ✔ **Nicotine Anonymous** is a 12-step program. To find out more, call 1-415-750-0328 or visit the Internet at `www.nicotine-anonymous.org`.

Relating Alcohol to High Blood Pressure

Now, this section tackles the second-most lethal thing that you can put into your body: alcohol. Or maybe it's the *most* lethal. I guess it depends on whether you specialize in lungs or livers. (In this section, I'm addressing people who drink more than a glass or two of wine a day and more than ten glasses a week.)

Alcohol raises blood pressure. Comparing the blood pressure of heavy drinkers (men who drink more than ten and women who drink more than five alcoholic beverages per week) with moderate drinkers and those who don't drink, shows that alcohol does indeed raise blood pressure. When non-drinkers drink alcohol, their blood pressure rises, and when heavy drinkers stop drinking, their blood pressure falls.

Abruptly stopping alcohol may cause a rise in blood pressure, so a doctor must monitor this carefully.

Drinking large quantities of alcohol in one sitting also raises blood pressure, but it returns to normal if the drinking doesn't continue. However, an individual who drinks excessively for extended periods of time has a persistent increase in blood pressure. The longer a person drinks, the higher the blood pressure.

It doesn't hurt to reemphasize that stopping one bad habit may ease the stopping of another. Cigarettes and alcohol go together like Fred Astaire and Ginger Rogers, but smoking and drinking isn't graceful or charming. Between 80 to 95 percent of alcoholics smoke cigarettes. Eliminating the power of one goes a long way towards eliminating the power of the other.

Considering the effects of alcoholism

Alcoholism, defined as the habitual or compulsive consumption of alcoholic liquor to excess, is an inherited physical abnormality, an inborn condition related to a certain type of body chemistry. Alcoholism is *not* a moral weakness.

A major medical consequence of alcoholism is the occurrence of brain attacks at a much higher rate. A study in *Stroke* (May 1998) showed that drinking four beers or the equivalent on a daily basis led to a considerable increase in brain attacks, even more that the increase in brain attacks caused by heavy smoking (more than 20 cigarettes daily).

If you're taking medication for high blood pressure and drinking heavily at the same time, you need to determine if you're an alcoholic to clarify the role of your drinking in your blood pressure.

You may be an alcoholic if you answer yes to two or more of the following questions: Have you . . .

- ✔ Tried to reduce your drinking?
- ✔ Felt angry when someone talked to you about your drinking?
- ✔ Felt guilty about drinking?
- ✔ Used alcohol in the morning to "start the day" and settle your nerves?

Another way to determine if you're an alcoholic is to count the number of drinks that you consume in a week. (A drink is a 12-ounce bottle of beer, 5 ounces of wine, or 1½ ounces of hard liquor.) Alcoholic men usually consume 15 or more drinks per week, and alcoholic women consume 12 or more. Those who consume more than five drinks in one sitting at least once a week are also considered alcoholics. Usually, alcoholics also . . .

- ✔ **Crave alcohol.**

  They have a strong need to drink.
- ✔ **Lose control when they drink.**

  They can't stop after they start.
- ✔ **Have a physical dependence on alcohol.**

  They have withdrawal symptoms if they don't drink.
- ✔ **Have a tolerance to alcohol.**

  They need more alcohol than a nonalcoholic individual to achieve the same level of inebriation.

The dire effects of demon drink

Endorphins, chemicals in the brain, are internal pleasure givers. The brain increases its release of endorphins when you drink alcohol. Similarly, habit-forming drugs, such as heroin, also stimulate increased production of endorphins, producing a feeling of euphoria. Although alcoholics require more alcohol than a heroin addict requires heroin to get the same "high," most people feel "high" at a blood level of .05 percent alcohol. The intoxication is severe at .2 percent blood level while at .3 percent, the drinker may be in a coma. Death may occur when the level is .35 percent or higher.

Who's drinking and how much?

Alcohol abuse can lead to two major long-term medical problems:

- Cirrhosis of the liver with liver failure
- Heart disease associated with high blood pressure

According to the *Journal of Studies on Alcohol* (November 2001), alcohol use begins in high school even though it's illegal to drink alcohol before the age of 18 in some states and 21 in the rest. In the last month, probably 70 percent of high school seniors have had alcohol to drink.

In the United States, the prevalence of alcoholism is 10 to 15 people per hundred, meaning that more than 10 million alcoholics are in this country. An additional 10 million are problem drinkers who may become alcoholics, and the number of male alcoholics is only slightly greater than the number of females.

Alcohol abuse costs the United States 116 billion dollars every year due to lost productivity, early death, medical treatment, and legal fees for all the problems alcoholics get themselves into.

Alcohol's other consequences

The following list of health consequences from excessive alcohol use is long. Unfortunately, you don't get one or another of these complications, but all of them at the same time. The load is heavy enough for anyone to bear but particularly for the elderly.

- Depression of the central nervous system with loss of ability to perform complex tasks, such as driving; decreased attention span and short-term memory; impaired motor coordination

- Degeneration of the brain with loss of coordination and emotional instability, and nerve degeneration with severe pain

- Addiction to tranquilizers to treat the emotional instability

- Physical damage in motor-vehicle crashes

- Increased risk of suicide and homicide

- Increased risk of unplanned pregnancy and sexually-transmitted diseases

- Giving birth to a baby with fetal-alcohol syndrome, stunted growth, mental retardation, and other abnormalities of the face and heart

- Poor nutrition from an irritated liver and intestinal tract, which produces heartburn, nausea, and gas

- Alcoholic heart disease

- Loss of sex drive

- Neglect of food intake and physical appearance

- Sleep loss

- Severe inflammation of the pancreas with severe abdominal pain and nausea

- Cirrhosis of the liver with gastrointestinal bleeding, liver failure, and death

- Increased incidence of cancer

Cancers of the mouth, throat, and esophagus occur more frequently among those who drink and smoke than among those who only drink or those who only smoke. The combination of drinking and smoking greatly increases the risk of cancer. A drinker is six times more likely to get mouth and throat cancer as compared to a nondrinker. A smoker is seven times more likely to get mouth and throat cancer as compared to a nonsmoker. But the individual who drinks and smokes is 38 times more likely to have mouth and throat cancer than the individual who neither drinks nor smokes.

Gaining by restraining

All the medical consequences of alcoholism start to reverse after you give up alcohol, particularly, for our purposes, the blood pressure. Cirrhosis of the liver, however, is irreversible after it occurs. In addition, you may regain your job, your family, and other loved ones, and your self-respect.

Through the years, the study of alcoholism and its treatment has proven useful in many ways. First of all, the more help that the alcoholic gets and uses, the greater the chance for prolonged sobriety. Specifically:

- ✔ Only 4 percent of alcoholics who try quitting on their own are sober after a year.
- ✔ 50 percent of alcoholics who go through treatment are sober after a year.
- ✔ 70 percent of alcoholics who go through treatment and regularly attend Alcoholics Anonymous are sober after a year.
- ✔ 90 percent of alcoholics who go through treatment, attend Alcoholics Anonymous, and go to aftercare once a week are sober after one year.

Treatment and follow-up after treatment is undoubtedly valid and important. Treatment consists of a brief intervention, during which the alcoholic is convinced to undergo therapy to stop drinking, and then a period of total abstinence from alcohol called *detoxification,* followed by techniques that keep the alcoholic sober for the rest of her life. These techniques include drugs and Alcoholics Anonymous.

A major step that the alcoholic can take is to join Alcoholics Anonymous (AA) Letting AA explain itself is probably best. I can tell you that more than 1 million recovered alcoholics are in AA in the United States and another million are in other countries. AA members meet in groups, large and small, to support one another. About 51,000 AA groups meet in the United States, and one can be found near you. Check online at www.alcoholics-anonymous.org or write to the main office to find a support group near you: Alcoholics Anonymous, Grand Central Station, P.O. Box 459, New York, NY 10163.

The intervention

The intervention refers to the steps that you can take to help the person who drinks excessively to stop while helping his loved ones to deal with the issues his drinking has created. Going through this process has been shown to be the best way to help all concerned. Even if the drinker can't be helped to stop, the other involved people benefit greatly.

- ✔ **Taking care of yourself.**

  If you are the partner, child, parent, or employer of an alcoholic, first help yourself by going to Al-Anon (a support program similar to Alcoholics Anonymous established for the loved ones of the alcoholic) and getting the support of a counselor. Only with the clear vision of an outside helper can you understand what you have to do to help the alcoholic.

✔ **Using outside help for the alcoholic.**

Find an addictions counselor to help you with the complicated process of getting your loved one or yourself off of alcohol.

✔ **Creating an intervention team.**

This team is made up of people who care about the alcoholic but whose lives have been made miserable at times by the former actions of the alcoholic. The addictions counselor is an important part of the team. Each person should tell the alcoholic in writing how she has made their lives miserable. They should tell the alcoholic to go to a treatment center and clearly indicate that they will no longer protect the alcoholic from her bad behaviors. They should clearly state how they will separate themselves from the alcoholic if treatment is not sought. For example, the spouse will leave the marriage.

✔ **Performing the intervention.**

When the alcoholic is sober, the intervention is carried out and not stopped until the alcoholic agrees to treatment or the professional feels that nothing further can be done.

Detoxification

Detoxification means complete abstinence from alcohol. During detoxification, the alcoholic must stop all drinking. Alcohol withdrawal consists of sweating and a rapid heartbeat, agitation, confusion, nausea and vomiting, and sometimes tremors or seizures. The alcoholic often becomes depressed. The doctor treats these symptoms with medications to control them. They may last three to seven days.

During detoxification, the alcoholic should be evaluated for his addiction's medical consequences, such as liver disease and abnormalities of blood clotting. Evidence of nutritional deficiencies is often found and should be treated with vitamins, minerals, and a healthy, balanced diet.

Can moderate drinking benefit your health?

For years, people thought that a drink a day would keep the doctor away. And a number of studies have shown that people who drink moderately (no more than two drinks daily for men and one for women) have improvements in the health of their heart and a lower rate of death than people who don't drink at all.

But a more recent study of 5,500 men in Scotland published in the *British Medical Journal* (June 1999) showed that drinking two drinks daily led to a higher risk of dying from all causes as compared with men who drank less alcohol. In another study from Harvard Medical School, a fat increase was discovered in the livers of men who ate well but had a daily dose of alcohol not large enough to cause inebriation. So a word to the wise: Don't start drinking to obtain the medical "benefits" of alcohol.

The long-term program

Total abstinence from alcohol is the goal of treatment. Absolutely no amount of alcohol, no matter how small, is acceptable.

The alcoholic enters a rehabilitation program of counseling, education, medical care, and nursing. Many of the people who help the alcoholic are recovering alcoholics who have "been there."

Medications are used to prevent the alcoholic from returning to drinking or to block the effects of alcohol. The principal medications in current use are

- **Disulfiram** (brand name *Antabuse*): When mixed with alcohol, Antabuse triggers a severe hangover — headache, nausea, vomiting, increased blood pressure, and a rapid heartbeat. The person taking disulfiram must be vigilant because many prepared foods, such as sauces and vinegars, contain alcohol, which can set off a reaction. Antabuse may continue to work up to two weeks after the individual quits taking it and shouldn't be used during pregnancy. Disulfiram also interacts with certain other medications, especially blood thinners and anticonvulsants, so your doctor must be aware of everything you're taking. It can negatively affect mental illness, cause a severe allergic skin reaction, and cause drowsiness in some people who shouldn't use dangerous machinery or drive a car while on disulfiram. It may also reduce sex drive. The medication is used as long as necessary until the patient is in control of his drinking. This may take months or even years.

- **Naltrexone** (brand name *Revia*): Naltrexone affects the pleasure chemicals that alcohol releases. The individual can no longer get high from alcohol, so there is little point in drinking. People don't become dependent on naltrexone and don't become euphoric when it's taken. Naltrexone has been known to cause dizziness, headache, and weight loss, and there are cases of naltrexone abuse. Individuals with severe liver or kidney damage shouldn't take naltrexone. It doesn't make a person sober nor does it prevent a person from enjoying other sources of pleasure. Naltrexone also blocks the effects of opiods, such as morphine. So if pain medication is needed, it must be a non-narcotic. Patients usually continue on naltrexone for three months if they stop drinking successfully.

- **Isradipine** (brand name *Dynacirc*): This is another drug that works by taking away the pleasure associated with drinking. It was originally used for the treatment of high blood pressure and found to help those people who were drinking heavily. The craving for alcohol rapidly diminishes and continues to decline as treatment continues. It may make you feel light-headed and dizzy, so driving should be avoided until you determine your reaction to it. It also causes headache and shouldn't be taken during pregnancy.

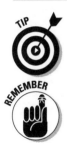

Using two of the drugs together may be more effective than one alone.

These drugs won't work on a long-term basis without a treatment program such as Alcoholics Anonymous.

Attending Alcoholics Anonymous

The support of AA is tremendously helpful for the alcoholic who utilizes it. A typical meeting consists of the group leader's description of the AA program followed by the personal histories of several members. A collection for the cost of the facilities and snacks is taken up and then the members leave or meet informally. All opinions and interpretations are those of the speaker himself. No one speaks for the whole group.

Alcoholics Anonymous provides an abundance of helpful literature, some of which is free and some is sold for a nominal fee. The success of AA is based on the power of one recovered alcoholic to help an uncontrolled drinker by passing along his experience and sobriety. This is done through the famous "Twelve Steps of Alcoholics Anonymous," which can be found in any of their publications.

Locating useful resources

Numerous resources are available to the alcoholic who wishes to recover if only she makes use of them. Some are listed below in no particular order. If you have access, you can find tons of information on the Internet. If not, call the phone number I've added to each resource.

- ✔ **The Internet Alcohol Recovery Center** is a central source for information on every aspect of alcohol abuse and treatment. A service of the University of Pennsylvania Health System, it has links to numerous resources and is a great place to start your education (after you've read my book, of course). It has such useful features as a substance abuse library and a directory of treatment professionals and support groups. You can call them at 215-243-9959 or find them online at `www.uphs.upenn.edu/recovery/index.html`.

- ✔ **Alcoholics Anonymous** has numerous sites on the Internet because so many of these groups dot the planet, but the central Web site is `www.alcoholics-anonymous.org`. Most of their publications are online along with directions to their groups worldwide. This is a key resource for anyone who lives with an alcoholic or is trying to quit alcohol. You can also call them at 212-870-3400.

✔ **The American Council on Alcoholism** is a national nonprofit organization dedicated to addressing alcoholism as a treatable disease through identification, education, intervention, and referral. They have useful links to sites concerning college drinking, drunk driving, general information on alcoholism, government resources, professional organizations that deal with alcoholism, treatment and recovery links, and links to drugs that help, and to the Web sites of the alcohol industry. It may be found on the Internet at www.aca-usa.org. Their site answers any question that you may have about alcoholism, or you can call them at 800-527-5344.

✔ **Al-Anon/Alateen** provides help for the victims (loved ones?) of the alcoholic. It uses the principles of AA to help these people to regain control over their lives and to see what action they can take to help the alcoholic. You find information on meetings, resources, and plenty of other help. Look for them at www.al-anon.alateen.org. You can also call 888-425-2666.

✔ **Mothers Against Drunk Driving** is another nationwide organization that provides information. It has over 600 chapters in this country and is dedicated to finding effective solutions to drunk driving and underage driving. Find them at www.madd.org/madd/aboutus. Their phone number is 800-438-6233.

Getting High on Caffeine

Caffeine is a chemical compound that's found in the leaves, seeds, and fruits of more than 63 plant species but most commonly comes from coffee and cocoa beans, cola nuts, and tea leaves. Coffee isn't the only source of caffeine. A can of cola contains 45 mg. Green tea contains 30 mg of caffeine. An ounce of chocolate has 20 mg in it. Even Anacin comes in at 65 mg for two tablets.

While the case against caffeine isn't nearly as tidy as that against tobacco and alcohol, no matter what form it's taken in, caffeine has been shown to temporarily raise blood pressure. Although a cup or two of coffee doesn't seem to be damaging over the long-term, our current tendency to drink multiple cups of "high octane" (heavily caffeinated) coffee is a definite cause of a persistent elevation in blood pressure. People who drink four to five cups of coffee daily have an increase in blood pressure of 5 mm Hg. (See Chapter 2 for more on blood pressure measurement.) If they continue to drink the same amount, the blood pressure may fall if they don't have high blood pressure already. If they do, they may be more sensitive to the blood pressure-raising effect of caffeine, and their blood pressure rise is sustained. This is particularly true of the elderly population.

A 5 mm Hg rise in blood pressure may sound trivial, but it results in a 21 percent rise in the incidence of heart disease and a 34 percent increase in the incidence of brain attacks (see Chapter 7). In addition, when combined with alcohol and/or tobacco, which is so often the case, it greatly increases the blood pressure-raising effect of those drugs.

Having a cup of coffee just before having your blood pressure measured is unwise. The acute elevation in blood pressure may convince your doctor that you have sustained high blood pressure.

How much is too much?

Who doesn't drink coffee with caffeine? Me. Several years ago, I stopped drinking caffeinated beverages and thus immediately stopped having abdominal pain, and I've had no abdominal pain since then. Otherwise, many people drink caffeine and plenty of it.

An ordinary cup of coffee has 100 mg of caffeine. A tall (12 ounce) cup of coffee at a nice café or fancy coffee shop has 375 mg, while a coffee grande has 550 mg. A short (8 ounce) cup of coffee contains 250 mg. You can see where a few cups of coffee can quickly add up to much more than the recommended maximum of 300 mg.

Caffeine and other health consequences

Caffeine is a mildly addictive drug. When a person stops drinking it, she will have withdrawal symptoms:

- ✔ Feelings of sleepiness
- ✔ Feelings of being overtired
- ✔ A severe headache

Caffeine also has a number of potential medical consequences when taken in large doses (over 300 mg daily) over a period of years:

- ✔ Thinning of the bone called *osteoporosis*

    Calcium is lost in the urine as a result of the urine-promoting effect of caffeine. Women (and men) are encouraged to manage this problem by taking milk with the caffeine and getting extra calcium from other sources.

- Infertility, birth defects, and miscarriages
- Heartburn (take it from me) and even ulcers due to increased stomach acid production
- When unfiltered (which was true of coffee before 1975), it increased the rate of heart disease.
- It may worsen premenstrual pain and increase formation of breast lumps, but this is controversial.
- It causes poor quality sleep and difficulty falling asleep.

Caffeine can keep you awake, but it does not improve your performance of complex tasks.

What you gain by giving up caffeine

Besides eliminating another unnecessary drug from your body, when you give up caffeine you eliminate the chance of developing any of the conditions in the preceding "Caffeine and other health consequences" section while helping to keep your blood pressure under control. As a woman, you may greatly enhance your chance of becoming pregnant and having a healthy pregnancy and delivery.

The coffee bean isn't a vegetable. You get no credit in the vegetable area of your DASH diet (see Chapter 9) for consuming it.

Warning: You could become a coffee addict if you name your child "Mocha" and your dog "Java."

Avoiding the beans, the chocolate, and the soda

If you consume caffeine in the form of no more than two cups of coffee daily, you should have no problem switching to decaffeinated drinks and avoiding other sources of caffeine, such as chocolate. I was in that category when I gave up caffeine, yet I did go through a period of mild withdrawal symptoms.

For the person who takes in much more in the form of giant cups of coffee or many cans of soda daily, the process of quitting caffeine may be more difficult. Here are some practical suggestions:

✔ Try to determine how much caffeine you're taking in each day. Check all foods and medications to make sure you're not missing an unexpected source.

✔ Reduce your intake and see how you feel as you withdraw.

✔ Gradually reduce your daily caffeine by 50 mg or so until you're free of it.

✔ Use exercise to give you the energy that you believe was coming from caffeine.

✔ Avoid the other habits that go with drinking coffee, such as smoking.

✔ Ask the people you live and eat with to help you by reducing their caffeine intake as well. The improvement they feel will make them grateful.

Using resources

You can check a few Internet sites for the latest information on this controversial drug. Among the best are

✔ **The Center for Science in the Public Interest** is a large Web source of information on exactly what its title suggests. They publish the Nutrition Action Healthletter. As new information on the health effects of caffeine becomes available, you can find it at this site with the address . Their phone number is 202-332-9110.

✔ Numerous university hospital sites are available on the Internet where you can search for information on caffeine. One of the best is Columbia University's Health Question & Answer Internet Service called "Go Ask Alice." It may be found at www.goaskalice.columbia.edu. This is an Internet site, so no phone number is given.

Some pros and cons of caffeine

The final determination on all the effects of coffee, negative and positive, isn't in. Some studies indicate that coffee may protect against cancer of the large intestine and rectum. Others suggest that it may have a protective effect against the damage that alcohol does to the liver. Very careful future studies can show whether this is valid.

But one proven damaging consequence of caffeine is that it affects the woman who wants to become pregnant. Consuming more than three cups of coffee with caffeine each day seems to reduce fertility. And the woman who is pregnant may deliver an underweight baby if she consumes more than three cups daily during her pregnancy. A few women who consumed enormous amounts of caffeine — up to 8 to 25 cups of coffee every day — delivered babies with birth defects.

Chapter 12

Exercising Your Way to Lower Blood Pressure

*W*hen I see new patients with high blood pressure, I give them a bottle of pills right away. But the pills aren't for oral consumption. Rather, they're for dropping on the floor and picking up one at a time several times a day — a good start to an exercise program.

You must make up your mind to exercise. Did you think you were given all those muscles just to cushion your bones? Exercise can lower blood pressure — especially the blood pressure of those who have high blood pressure. The benefits of a regular exercise program can't be denied. Lowering your blood pressure is just one of the many reasons for committing yourself to a regular exercise program. Exercise also causes weight reduction and weight loss maintenance, which also helps to lower blood pressure.

An exercise test can also help find out the people who need to be observed for the development of high blood pressure. Those who have an exaggerated rise in blood pressure during exercise are much more likely to develop sustained high blood pressure later in life. They need to be watched more carefully.

I asked a patient who refused to exercise whether it was because of ignorance or apathy. The patient replied, "I don't know, and I don't care." Read this chapter. Then if you don't exercise, it won't be because of ignorance at least.

Understanding How Physical Activity Benefits Your Heart and Body

Exercise strengthens all the muscles that are involved in the movement. If you walk or jog, your leg muscles are strengthened. If you lift packages, your arm muscles are strengthened. Whatever the exercise, your heart muscles are made stronger. At the same time, your body opens up your arteries to allow for more flow of nutrients into the tissues. The combination of a stronger, more efficient heart and more open blood vessels leads to lowering blood pressure.

Lowering your blood pressure is a good enough reason to make exercise an important part of your lifestyle, but if you need more reasons, check out the listing that follows for some of what exercise can do for you.

- Improve your memory
- Reduce the risk of breast cancer and large intestinal cancer
- Lowers blood sugar, thus protecting you against diabetes
- Increases energy level
- Improves mood
- Makes you sexier
- Helps you sleep better
- Strengthens your bones
- Lowers bad cholesterol and raises good cholesterol

Could you possibly need any more reasons? If you do, pick up a copy of *Fitness For Dummies,* 2nd Edition, by Suzanne Schlosberg and Liz Neporent, MA (Wiley), where you find 100 reasons to become fit.

Preparing for Exercise

You need to take three important steps before you begin an exercise program. First, determine your current physical condition to decide what type of exercise program is right for your current fitness level. Second, choose the exercises that you plan to make part of your program. And finally, get the right equipment.

Checking your physical condition

Before you start an exercise program, find out the level of your fitness at the beginning, so that you have something to use to chart your progress. One simple way to test your fitness level is to take your pulse, walk a mile, and note the time that it takes you as well as your pulse rate at the end of the mile. The time and your pulse give you have a baseline from which to compare as you improve.

To take your pulse, place your index and middle finger over the artery in the wrist that's about ½ inch in from the outside of the wrist when it's facing with the palm upward. (Don't use your thumb to feel because it has its own pulse and can confuse your count). Count the number of beats for 15 seconds and multiply by four to get your one-minute pulse rate. If you can't feel your pulse in the wrist, try feeling the pulse in your neck where it's much stronger. Write down the number before you forget it! You can do this simple test about once a month and you'll be astounded at your progress as your pulse gets slower and slower — indicating a much more efficient heart.

If you haven't exercised for many years, don't start a program without some preparation. If you're over the age of 40, you should talk to your doctor and have a physical examination. Your doctor may recommend an *exercise electrocardiogram,* better known as an exercise test or a stress test. The test looks at the response of your heart to fairly vigorous exercise. If you get through an exercise electrocardiogram without problems such as chest pain, severe shortness of breath, or changes in your electrocardiogram, you're probably in good enough shape to begin an exercise program.

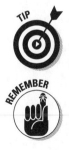

Ask your doctor to help you map out an exercise plan that can achieve your goal of strengthening your heart and preventing high blood pressure. If you've already been diagnosed with high blood pressure, discuss a plan that can help lower your blood pressure to an agreeable level.

When you begin your exercise program, start slowly and build up over time. You don't need to rush to get to a certain level of exercise by a certain date. Gradually work your way along until you achieve your goal. You also don't need to go farther and faster after you reach a level of fitness that affects your blood pressure. That desired fitness level may lower your blood pressure by as much as 10 millimeters of mercury systolic (see Chapter 2) — a lowering that's as good as most pills can accomplish. Going farther and faster, however, won't get you much lower than that. If you're really *enjoying* the exercise and *want* to rev it up, that's up to you, but don't think that doing so can further lower your blood pressure.

Choosing exercises

For maximum fitness, most exercise programs combine two types of exercises: aerobic and anaerobic.

- ✔ **Aerobic** means "with oxygen." During aerobic exercise, the body uses oxygen to help provide energy. Aerobic activities can be sustained for more than a few minutes and involve major groups of muscles, particularly the legs but also the arms if you can't use your legs. These activities, such as walking, running, cycling, tennis, basketball, and so forth, get your heart to pump faster during the exercise.

- ✔ **Anaerobic** means "without oxygen." Anaerobic exercises are brief and very intense. They can't be sustained for very long and depend on sources of energy that are already available. Examples are lifting heavy weights and doing the 100-yard dash.

Engaging in a regular aerobic exercise program can, over time, lower your blood pressure up to 10 millimeters of mercury systolic and enable you to get off a blood pressure medication. Anaerobic exercises, although great for increasing the strength of individual muscles, don't go on long enough to improve heart function or lower your blood pressure. But a program of both aerobic and anaerobic exercises gives you the best of both worlds — lower blood pressure and stronger muscles. (See the "Exercising for Strength" section later in this chapter for practical anaerobic exercise ideas.)

The range of aerobic exercise choices is limitless. Mix it up a bit. Play tennis several days a week and do something else, perhaps walking, the other days. Walking is the exercise that almost everybody can do. You don't have to belong to a special club to walk. Unless you live in an area that has snow a good portion of the year, you can walk outside most any day — even in the rain. (Use an umbrella; you won't melt.) You can easily walk alone or with another person. Walking with a friend makes the activity more pleasant and also causes you both to encourage each other to stay committed to exercising regularly.

Table 12-1 is a walking program that can get you up to speed eventually but that starts slow enough so that most people can complete the first part without a great deal of difficulty. If the distance is too great for you, begin with half the distance and work your way up until you've accomplished each level once each day for seven days. Don't move to the next level before you've done the previous level seven times.

If you did the test described earlier in this chapter to evaluate your fitness, you already know how fast you can do a mile. Start at that level, not a slower level. If you didn't do a fitness test, begin the seven days at the level that you can do the first time that you try.

Table 12-1 breaks down the walking program into 15 different levels so that you can work your way up to a desired level of fitness to lower your blood pressure. Start at the highest one that you can do now and build from there.

Table 12-1	Walking Program to Achieve Lower Blood Pressure	
Level	**Distance (in miles)**	**Time (in minutes)**
1	1	30
2	1	28
3	1	26
4	1	24
5	1	22
6	1	20
7	1½	32
8	1½	31
9	1½	30
10	1½	29
11	1½	28
12	1½	27
13	1½	26
14	1½	25
15	1½	24

You must complete one level seven times before moving on to the next level.

When you reach the last level, you can stay at that level permanently. You'll have an acceptable workout that'll make a significant difference in your blood pressure as well as other aspects of your health. Surely you can spare less than half an hour daily to make a huge impact on your health.

Walking is great exercise, and certainly one of the simplest, but don't feel like you *have* to walk to enjoy the pressure-lowering effects of exercise. If you prefer to do some other types of aerobic activities, feel free! Just make sure that you choose aerobically effective activities that you're able to do and able to stick with. Some other kinds of exercise that you may like to do are shown in Table 12-2 later in this chapter. In addition, consider racquetball, squash, handball, rowing, judo, karate, social dancing, and singles tennis. People from different cultures may also have different exercises that they particularly like, such as soccer, rugby, and cricket. *What* you do doesn't really matter; you just have to be sure to do *something*.

Getting the right equipment

If you plan to engage in an exercise that may cause friction in your joints, such as walking and jogging, get the best footwear that you can afford. Some of the sneakers that are available seem awfully pricey, but when you consider what you save in the "long run" (pun intended) in health costs, then they're well worth the price.

Try to find a store where the staff is knowledgeable about shoe needs, perhaps one that caters to runners and walkers.

Make sure that you have the right clothes for your exercise. Dressing in layers is a good idea because you can remove clothing as you heat up. Some sports clothes are better than others in that they "sweat," allowing your perspiration to pass through and evaporate rather than sticking to your body. This will both cool you off and help you to feel less "wet" as you exercise. Cotton isn't a good choice because it absorbs the moisture and holds it against your skin. One of the polyesters works well. For cooler weather, choose an outer layer that repels wind and rain but allows sweat to pass through.

If you choose to do plenty of biking, make sure that you have a bike that's suitable for the terrain where you plan to ride. Bikes that are good for flat streets are very different from mountain bikes. Even the tires are different. If you want to limit yourself to an indoor stationary cycle, make sure that the quality is good. Plenty of resources, such as *Consumer Reports,* are available. And you can also find help on the Internet. One Web site, "What's the Best Bike" (www.whatsthebest-bike.com), can help you with your choices.

Other resources are available to help you with the choice of exercise equipment, such as treadmills and weight machines. You might start with an article called "Purchasing a Treadmill" that can be found on the Web at www.primusweb.com/fitnesspartner/library/equipment/treadmil.htm.

Knowing How Much to Do

People with high blood pressure have a post-exercise fall in blood pressure that may last seven or eight hours. Therefore, *daily* exercise can have a much more profound effect on your blood pressure than exercise that's done only three or four times a week.

You want to know whether your exercise is making a difference in your fitness. You could do a fitness test each time, but that's not a good idea because you won't make huge strides each time that you exercise, and you'll definitely be disappointed. For many years, fitness advisors suggested that you measure your heart rate during exercise. Using a simple formula, you could determine if your pulse fell into a range called "the training range" that was fast enough to improve your fitness but not too fast to overexert your heart. Now it's known that the concept of the training range is probably not useful.

People can exercise with a faster pulse than their training range and benefit from it. Instead, rate your physical activity of choice according to the Perceived Exertion Scale to determine if the activity is making a difference in your fitness. To use this scale, rate the degree of your exertion while performing a certain activity from being very, very light to being very, very hard — according to your personal physical ability level. In between are very light, fairly light, somewhat hard, hard, and very hard. If you exercise to the level of very hard, you're doing the amount of exercise that's most beneficial. Keep in mind that as your fitness level increases, your definition of very hard changes. What was once very hard may become fairly light. Very hard exercise also corresponds to a level at which you start having trouble talking comfortably.

Exercise is beneficial for every stage of high blood pressure (see Chapter 2). However, doctors generally recommend that people with blood pressure in the higher stages 2 and 3, where the blood pressure is greater than 160 systolic and 100 diastolic, do their exercise at a slightly lower level than stage 1 patients. Referring to the Perceived Exertion Scale, stage 2 and 3 patients should work at a level of "somewhat hard" rather than "very hard."

Exercising to Lose Weight

Exercise can help you lose weight. If you expect to lose weight as you exercise, you need to exercise at least six days a week for at least 30 minutes each time.

A pound of fat contains 3,500 *kilocalories* (kcals). A kilocalorie is a measurement of energy, specifically the amount of energy needed to raise the temperature of a kilogram of water 1 degree centigrade. To lose a pound of fat, you must do at least 3,500 kilocalories of exercise greater than the number of kilocalories that you eat. For example, if you eat 2,000 kilocalories each day to maintain your weight, doing 500 kilocalories of exercise daily more than you usually do causes a weight loss of a pound in seven days (500 times 7 equals 3,500). Doing only 250 kilocalories of extra exercise takes 14 days to lose the same pound. An hour of walking daily, which burns 4 kilocalories per minute, results in 240 kilocalories of energy loss daily.

Table 12-2 shows the number of kilocalories that you burn doing several different kinds of exercise for 30, 45, or 60 minutes.

Table 12-2	Kilocalories Burned Doing Various Exercises		
Activity	*30 minutes*	*45 minutes*	*60 minutes*
Aerobic dance	342	513	684
Basketball	282	423	564
Bicycling (12 mph)	283	425	566
Cross-country skiing	291	438	583
Golf (carrying your bag)	174	261	348
Running 10-min miles	365	549	732
Swimming	250	375	500
Doubles tennis	85	128	170
Walking 20-min mile on flat surface	120	180	240
Walking 20-min mile uphill	162	243	324
Walking 15-min mile on flat surface	146	219	292
Walking 15-min mile uphill	206	309	412
Water aerobics	140	210	280

Exercising for Strength

A complete exercise program includes both aerobic exercises to lower your blood pressure and anaerobic exercises to strengthen your muscles. Strengthening your muscles allows you to do more aerobic exercise as well as improve your balance. To add an anaerobic element to your workout, get yourself some *dumbbells* of various weights and some *barbells,* to which you can add progressively more weight as you get stronger.

If you have high blood pressure, you should use weight sizes that allow you to do many repetitions of an exercise instead of doing a few extreme lifts with very large weights. Extreme lifting may suddenly raise your blood pressure to unacceptable levels.

A weight lifting program requires no more than 15 minutes of your time about five days a week. Do it for two days, skip a day, for another three days, skip a day, then back to two days, and so on. These breaks allow your muscles to recover between exercise workouts.

Evaluating the strength of your upper and lower body

Count how many push-ups you can do to evaluate your upper-body strength. To do a push-up, lie face down on the floor with your palms about shoulder-width apart. Push yourself up off the floor, straightening your arms and keeping your back and legs straight. Lower yourself until your chest just touches the floor, but don't let your weight rest on the floor. Then push yourself up again. Count how many you can do before growing too tired.

Count the number of squats that you can do to evaluate your lower-body strength. To do a squat, stand up straight with your arms by your sides and legs about shoulder-width apart. Begin to bend your knees as you raise your arms to a horizontal position at your sides. When you have bent your knees so that your thighs are parallel with the ground, go back up again. Then repeat the movement. See how many you can do.

Save these numbers for future comparison. You want to test yourself at intervals of four to six weeks to keep track of your progress and keep yourself motivated to stay on the exercise program.

The following list describes seven exercises that can improve your upper-body strength. You can do these exercises in 15 minutes. Simply do 15 repetitions of each exercise and move on to the next. Each series of 15 repetitions of seven exercises is called a *circuit*. You should do two circuits without stopping each time that you exercise. Start with an amount of weight that allows you to complete the 15 repetitions. If you can't do 15, you're using too much weight and overexerting yourself.

- **Shoulder press:** Stand with your feet shoulder-width apart and knees slightly bent. With dumbbells in each hand, start with your hands next to your shoulders facing inward. Raise the dumbbells over your head until your arms are straight. Bring the weights back down to the starting position, palms facing each other.

- **Lateral raise:** Hold a dumbbell in each hand by your sides, palms facing each other. Raise the dumbbells out to the sides, keeping your arms straight (but don't lock your elbows) and your palms facing the floor, until they're above your head. Return them to the starting position.

- **Bent-over rowing:** Bend from the waist, keeping your knees slightly bent, until your upper body is parallel with the floor. With a dumbbell in each hand and your arms hanging straight down, slowly raise the dumbbells out to the side until they're in line with your shoulders. Lower them again.

- **Good mornings:** Stand straight with a single dumbbell held over your head by both hands. Keeping your arms straight over your head, bend from the waist until your torso and arms are parallel with the floor. Then raise yourself to the starting point.

- **Flys:** Lie on your back with one dumbbell in each hand and your arms opened out to each side at shoulder height. Slowly raise the dumbbells in over your body until they touch above your chest. Slowly lower them back to the starting position.

- **Pullovers:** Lie on your back with your knees bent, holding one dumbbell with both hands above your chest. Lower the dumbbell back over your head until it touches the floor. Then raise it back over your chest.

- **Curls:** Stand straight up, holding a barbell in each hand in front of you. With your palms facing out, slowly bend your elbows until your hands are shoulder height. Lower them back slowly to the starting position.

A couple of standard exercises for strengthening leg muscles include the following:

- To do a lunge, stand straight with your feet about shoulder-width apart. Hold a light dumbbell in each hand, palms facing your body. Take a long step forward with the right foot and bend the right leg until your thigh is parallel with the ground. Hold the position a second, and then step back and straighten your leg. Lunge forward with the other leg.

- A squat improves the strength of many different leg muscles. Begin by placing a barbell containing light weights behind your neck, holding it with your hands. Stand straight with your feet hip-width apart. Bend your knees slowly and squat until your thighs are parallel with the ground. Pause, and then rise to the standing position.

You'll be amazed and delighted at the rapid progress you make in terms of body strength, increased fitness, and increased self-assurance if you follow this simple program. Just be sure to increase the weights as they become easier to lift to continue reaping the rewards. Among other benefits, you'll

- Keep your bones stronger
- Prevent injuries by improving balance
- Look better
- Speed up your metabolism

You can expect to increase your strength anywhere from 7 to 40 percent after ten weeks of training your muscle groups.

Utilizing Other Types of Body Movement to Lower Your Blood Pressure

Although aerobic exercise is extremely helpful for lowering blood pressure, other disciplines can help accomplish this goal as well. So-called *alternative therapies* have been shown to reduce blood pressure. When combined with exercise, the result can be significant. You may want to consider trying one or several of these practices. They have some overlap in their effects, but each one is distinctive enough to have a following of devotees.

Yoga

Yoga is a series of postures and breathing exercises originally developed in India over 5,000 years ago as a way to achieve *union* (yoga) with the "divine consciousness." Today, people often practice Yoga as a way of improving their health and well-being without putting an emphasis on Yoga's religious side. Yoga attempts to unite your body and your mind, so that your mind can function better in a more healthy body.

Numerous studies have shown that Yoga can lower blood pressure. This effect persists as long as the practice continues, and it often disappears if the individual stops practicing Yoga.

Over the 5,000 years of Yoga's existence, it has evolved in many different directions as different teachers have developed their philosophies. As a result, Yoga has eight main branches. *Hatha Yoga,* the most popular branch, emphasizes physical fitness more than the others. But this branch subscribes to plenty of meditation and spiritualism as well.

An excellent source of information about all aspects of Yoga is *Yoga For Dummies,* by Georg Feuerstein, PhD, and Larry Payne, PhD (Wiley). I highly recommend it to you. The Internet also offers many excellent Yoga sites. The following are two of the best:

- ✔ **The Yoga Site** (www.yogasite.com) can answer all your questions and direct you to many other useful sites.

- ✔ **The Yoga Directory** (www.yogadirectory.com) directs you to any type of service that you may need that has to do with Yoga from books and publications to centers and organizations, and from retreats and vacations to teachers and training.

Meditation

Meditation is a practice that involves concentrating on an object, a sound, a word, or the breath in order to diminish random thoughts. The result is a calmer, more peaceful mind. Some aspects of Yoga involve meditation, particularly the awareness of the breathing, but meditation doesn't involve the assumption of any specific body postures like Yoga does.

Many clinical studies have shown that meditation can lower the blood pressure and keep it down, as long as the practice is continued.

Just like Yoga, meditation has gone in different directions over the years of its existence. The most popular form is *Transcendental Meditation.* You can find out much more about this technique by obtaining (you guessed it) *Meditation For Dummies,* by Stephan Bodian (Wiley). Some of the best Internet resources on meditation are the following:

- ✔ **Learning Meditation** (www.learningmeditation.com) is an award-winning site that explains what meditation is all about and how you can use it in your daily life to find more calm and serenity. The author of this site actually prefers the term *conscious relaxation* or *chosen relaxation* to meditation. The site is well done, and I highly recommend it.

- ✔ **Holistic Online** (www.holisticonline.com) describes just about every kind of alternative therapy that exists, including meditation and even humor therapy. If meditation isn't what you're looking for, the site probably has something else that you can get into.

Hypnosis

Hypnosis is a form of *guided meditation* (guided by another person or oneself) that slows down the brain and allows the hypnotized person to respond, within limitations, to the suggestions of the hypnotist. A hypnotized person won't do anything that she doesn't want to do. The definition often describes a sleeplike state, but practitioners insist that the hypnotized person isn't asleep because she can hear and respond.

Hypnosis has been shown to lower blood pressure when appropriate relaxation instructions are given. People can hypnotize themselves and control blood pressure effectively.

You can find some excellent information on hypnosis on the Internet (what a surprise!). The Web sites that appear to have some very useful and valid information consist of the following:

- ✔ **Hypnosis.com** (www.hypnosis.com) has frequently asked questions that provide a clear explanation of what hypnosis is and what it can do for you. It clears up many myths about this useful therapy, particularly the myth that you can be induced to do something under hypnosis that you would never do ordinarily. These questions actually come from the newsgroup alt.hypnosis, and the answers are excellent.

- ✔ **The American Society of Clinical Hypnosis** Web site (www.asch.net) can help you find a therapist and explains what certification as a hypnotist is all about. It directs you to videos and books that help you to get a clearer picture of this technique.

Biofeedback

Biofeedback was developed in the late 1960s. It's a technique in which you train yourself, with the aid of *biofeedback machines,* to alter a so-called involuntary function, such as heart rate, body temperature, or in your case, blood pressure. (Biofeedback machines detect a person's internal bodily functions, so that the functions can be altered.) For the purposes of this discussion, the bodily function of interest is the blood pressure, and biofeedback can effectively lower blood pressure.

An example of a biofeedback technique is the use of a biofeedback machine that picks up electrical signals from muscles and translates them into a flashing light. In order to reduce the tension in muscles, the person using the machine figures out how to slow down the flashes of light. After awhile, the person no longer needs the machine to know when to relax and simply uses the methods to relax that she discovered *with* the machine. Biofeedback experiments show that people have more control over *involuntary bodily functions* than ever realized. Blood pressure happens to be one of these functions that can be altered.

Various kinds of equipment are available that you can use for biofeedback. Numerous Internet sites can help you find out about them. One of these sites is the Holistic Online site (www.holisticonline.com) mentioned in the "Meditation" section earlier in this chapter. A couple of others that can be of value for you are as follows:

- ✔ **The Association for Applied Psychophysiology and Biofeedback** Web site (www.aapb.org) contains answers to your questions as well as sources of practitioners, a bookstore for relevant books, and a source of links to more information.

- ✔ **The Biofeedback Network** (www.biofeedback.net) is an online source for equipment, information, links, practitioners, and biofeedback centers. Its mission is to provide "Quality On-line Biofeedback Resources to the world biofeedback community." That community may include you.

Yoga, meditation, hypnosis, and biofeedback are the most useful forms of alternative therapy for high blood pressure, but by no means are they the *only* forms. Holistic Online (www.holisticonline.com) lists no fewer than 20 different forms of alternative medicine. I can't vouch for the value of each form when it comes to treating high blood pressure, but people can follow many different paths toward controlling their blood pressure. Perhaps one of these methods will appeal to you, and you can utilize it to save yourself from years of medical problems and expenses related to high blood pressure (not to mention all the other diseases that are waiting out there for you).

Chapter 13

When Lifestyle Changes Don't Do It All: Drug Therapy

In This Chapter

▶ Getting a grip on drug features and categories

▶ Looking at what drugs expel water, salt, or potassium

▶ Comparing side effects

▶ Finding the drug that's right for you as an individual

▶ Recognizing brand names

*A*s I reviewed a recent publication on the treatment of high blood pressure with drugs, I came to a table listing the drugs that are currently available — no less than 57 different drugs in five different classes. Surely, a doctor could find one or more that would be perfect for you.

Not so fast! Have you done everything in your power to maximize the lifestyle changes that lower the blood pressure without drugs as discussed in Chapters 8 through 12? If you can say "Yes!" to this question and your blood pressure is still elevated, go ahead and ask your doctor about giving you a prescription for one of the drugs described in this chapter. If the answer is no, go back and do whatever you can to reduce your blood pressure without drugs.

The choices are limitless, but don't let every cute little new drug that comes along fool you. Designed to manipulate your imagination, glitzy TV and radio commercials and magazine ads suggest that your life can be a bowl of cherries if you pop a new drug. Some drugs are inappropriate for some people with high blood pressure and not others, and some drugs have miserable side effects — side effects that may affect you and just a few other people. Also, if you're already taking another prescription medicine, adding another drug could create a problem.

After I answer the general questions about drugs, I take up the individual drug classes and the drugs within them. You need to know how they act, how long they act, what the side effects are, what dosages you should take, how they interact with other medications, and what physical abnormalities you may have that preclude their use.

As I point out elsewhere in this book, despite the availability of excellent drugs, only about 25 percent of all people with high blood pressure control it. This brings up the problem of compliance. Taking your drug the first weeks or months after your doctor has made a diagnosis of high blood pressure is easy, but what about the years after that? As you continue to suffer from high blood pressure — the silent killer — will you lose your resolve to keep it controlled? After all, you may feel fine. You may not have seen your doctor for six months or a year. Of course, losing your resolve to control your blood pressure would be a serious mistake. However, your complete understanding of your medication as well as the reasons that you're taking it can help you to continue it. That's the reason for the high level of detail in this chapter.

Because you may be taking only one or two of the many drugs discussed in this chapter, you may confine your review to those drugs. But you should at least check the introductory remarks for each of the drug classes in this chapter. Your doctor may find that you would do much better if you started taking a prescription from another class. Take a look at the section on "Choosing a Drug" coming up later to make sure you're on the right track. Being an informed consumer can at least put you in a position to ask your doctor intelligent questions.

Your pharmacist can be a great resource for drug information. Also, a publication called the *Physicians' Desk Reference* (PDR) is available in most doctor's offices and hospital libraries. It has the latest information about all drugs.

Establishing Drug Characteristics

High blood pressure medications have different characteristics and features — some of which may be beneficial and some of which may be detrimental to you. Find out about a medication's main features before chasing a new pill down with a glass of water.

How effective is it?

Doctors like to have proof in the form of medical studies that the drugs are effective and that they work as advertised. This takes ten years or more after a drug has been approved by the Food and Drug Administration (FDA) and comes onto the market, and many of the drugs in this chapter have been around for only a few years. Drug manufacturers often claim that because a new drug belongs to the same class as a proven old drug, it should work the same. However, the new drug may produce side effects that only make themselves apparent after years of use on thousands of people. So you have to be wary.

How much can it lower blood pressure as compared to another drug?

Up to a certain point, the lower the blood pressure, the better off the patient. Several studies have shown that when the blood pressure is lowered below a certain level (which is not the same for each person), the risk of a heart attack increases, possibly because the pressure is so low that not enough blood is reaching the heart muscle. None of the commonly used drugs, when used alone, lower the blood pressure past that point. But of the various classes, thiazide diuretics lower the diastolic blood pressure about the same as other drugs, but the thiazide diuretics lower the systolic blood pressure more than the others.

Can two drugs that lower blood pressure to the same extent have the same effect on the disease and death that's caused by high blood pressure?

Thiazide diuretics lower blood pressure more than the other classes of commonly used drugs.

The evidence shows that even when a drug other than a thiazide diuretic lowers the blood pressure to the same extent, thiazides prevent disease and death more than other blood pressure-lowering drugs.

You may have concluded that I prefer thiazide diuretics for initial drug treatment for high blood pressure. Well, you're right!

Assuming that a blood pressure-lowering drug prevents the long-term consequences of high blood pressure is natural, but this isn't necessarily the case. But the old standards, especially the thiazide diuretics, have proven effective (though not in all circumstances).

The evidence shows that even when a drug other than a thiazide diuretic lowers the blood pressure to the same extent, thiazides prevent disease and death more than other drugs for high blood pressure. If you've concluded that I have a definite preference for thiazide diuretics as initial drug treatment for high blood pressure, you're right.

Presenting the Classes of Drugs

Drugs that lower blood pressure are divided into several different classes: diuretics, drugs that act on the nervous system, vasodilators, calcium channel blocking agents, angiotensin-converting enzyme inhibitors, and angiotensin II receptor blockers. Each class works by a different mechanism that I discuss later in this chapter.

The drugs in this chapter are discussed according to the way that they lower blood pressure. All the drugs currently available in each class are mentioned because your doctor may have a preference for one or another. The drugs are referred to by their generic name, the official chemical designation for that drug. Many manufacturers may make the same drug but give it their own brand name. The brand names are listed in parentheses after the generic name. Because you probably know the drug by its brand name, you can find an alphabetical listing of brand names at the end of this chapter. Then go to the correct generic drug (scientific name) to discover more about it.

Many of these drugs are available in drug combinations, which take advantage of the fact that two drugs of different classes are often more potent together than the sum of each one separately. The many drug combinations are listed by brand names at the end of the section to which they belong.

Diuretics

Of all the drug classes, the only one that has consistently reduced the illness and death associated with high blood pressure when it's the first treatment is the diuretic class and specifically the thiazide diuretics. See the "Thiazide and thiazidelike diuretic group" section later in this chapter for more on thiazide diuretics.

Diuretics, also known as "water pills," lower blood pressure by forcing the body to rid itself of salt and water through the kidneys into the urine. Depending on the place in the kidneys where they're active (see Chapter 6), diuretics rid the body of more or less salt and water. However, after a couple of months, the body overcomes the reduction in body fluids. At this point, it's a reduction in the resistance to blood flow that accounts for the ongoing fall in blood pressure. Depending on where the medication is acting along the nephron (see Chapter 6), diuretics are divided into different groups as follows:

- **Thiazide and thiazidelike diuretic group:** Although they're not the most effective drugs for ridding the body of excess salt and water, the most effective group for lowering blood pressure is the thiazide and thiazidelike diuretic group. This group acts at the distal tubule of the nephron (see Chapter 6) to cause the increased excretion of sodium and chloride.

- **Loop diuretics:** A second group, the loop diuretics, acts at the thick ascending limb of the loop of Henle (see Chapter 6), part of the filtering mechanism of the kidneys. These drugs have a potent effect on salt and water elimination.

- **Potassium-sparing diuretics:** A third group, the potassium-sparing diuretics function at the late distal tubule and the collecting tubule of the nephron (see Chapter 6). The result is only a mild increase in sodium excretion and chloride excretion but a tendency to reduce the excretion of potassium. Because the other diuretics cause potassium loss, the potassium-sparing diuretics are important for maintaining body potassium.

- **Aldosterone-antagonist group:** The final group of useful diuretics is the aldosterone-antagonist group. In the United States, only one is currently available, spironolactone. This group blocks the action of aldosterone, a natural hormone that causes salt and water retention. If its action is blocked, more salt and water is excreted into the urine while potassium loss is reduced. These drugs could be included in the potassium-sparing group, but they go about lowering blood pressure in an altogether different manner than the potassium-sparing group — they deactivate aldosterone.

Thiazide and thiazidelike diuretic group

Thiazide diuretics, the most effective blood pressure-lowering drugs, have been prescribed for more than 40 years and have the following positive characteristics:

- Can be taken once daily (an important issue in compliance with medication)

- Low cost

- Often as effective in low dosage as in higher dosage, thus reducing the problem of side effects

- Lowers the blood pressure about 15 mm Hg systolic and 7 mm Hg diastolic

- As compared with the other classes of drugs for high blood pressure, appears to be more tolerable because of the low rate with which people stop taking it

✔ Reduces the size of an enlarged heart (a sign of uncontrolled high blood pressure) about the same as the other classes of drugs

✔ Especially useful among African Americans and the elderly

Common side effects of thiazide diuretics include

✔ Initially induces sleep loss due to urination (but this side effect is offset by taking medication early in the day)

✔ Reduces calcium excretion in the urine and may provoke elevated blood calcium levels

✔ Not recommended during pregnancy and breast-feeding

✔ In higher dosage, causes excessive potassium loss, increases serum cholesterol, increases the body's resistance to its own insulin and a resultant increased intolerance to glucose, the sugar in the blood. In people with a tendency toward diabetes, use of thiazides may increase this tendency.

✔ Causes problems with erection in men, especially when used in higher dosages.

✔ Reduces the activity of certain other drugs, especially blood thinners (anticoagulants), drugs to reduce uric acid in the blood, antidiabetic drugs called *sulfonylureas* (drugs with names such as chlorpropamide, tolazamide, and tolbutamide) and insulin.

✔ Increases the activity of certain other drugs, particularly a heart drug called *digitalis,* and a drug called *lithium,* which is used for psychiatric impairment, and vitamin D.

The following sections look at individual drugs within the thiazide and thiazidelike diuretic group.

Hydrochlorothiazide

Of all the thiazide diuretics, hydrochlorothiazide (HydroDIURIL, Hydrochlorothiazide Capsules, Hydrochlorothiazide Oral Solution, Hydrochlorothiazide Tablets) is probably prescribed the most often. It has proved its value over many years and is known to be effective in small doses. However, hydrochlorothiazide isn't recommended for those with kidney failure or an allergic hypersensitivity to such drugs as sulfonamide antibiotics. This diuretic must also be used carefully in the presence of severe liver disease.

Some studies have shown that lower doses of hydrochlorothiazide actually reduce heart attacks more often than higher doses. If you're taking 50 mg of hydrochlorothiazide or even more for high blood pressure, ask your doctor to lower the dose to 25 mg to see if your blood pressure remains low. If so, try for 12.5 mg. The reduced frequency of side effects at this low dose makes such a trial worthwhile.

A higher dose of 50 mg is associated with potassium loss and increased blood sugar, but these side effects may be milder or disappear altogether at a lower dosage. If the blood glucose is extremely elevated, it may be necessary to discontinue the drug. To counter the loss of potassium, a potassium-sparing agent may be combined with hydrochlorothiazide because oral potassium isn't nearly as effective, and it's hard to take. (See more on these agents in the "Potassium-sparing diuretics" section coming up later in this chapter.)

See your doctor if you suffer from the following symptoms that suggest that you're losing too much potassium and body fluids:

- ✔ Confusion
- ✔ Drowsiness
- ✔ Dry mouth
- ✔ Muscle pains
- ✔ Nausea and vomiting
- ✔ Thirst
- ✔ Weakness

Hydrochlorothiazide comes in a 25 and a 50 mg pill. The recommended dosage is one 25 mg tablet daily, although starting with 12.5 mg, especially for an elderly person, is even better. It's taken once a day. Because it's eliminated from the body through the kidneys, it shouldn't be given when kidney failure is present.

Chlorothiazide

Chlorothiazide (Diuril Tablets, Diuril Oral Suspension, Chlorothiazide Tablets) is almost identical to hydrochlorothiazide. Because of a slight difference in the chemical makeup of chlorothiazide, it only has about a tenth of the potency of hydrochlorothiazide. It comes in 250 and 500 mg tablets.

All the information under hydrochlorothiazide pertains to this drug.

Bendroflumethiazide

Bendroflumethiazide (Naturetin) has a similar structure to hydrochlorothiazide, but it's ten times as strong. It shares the features of that drug, including the side effects. It comes as 5 and 10 mg tablets. The dose is usually 2.5 to 5 mg daily or on alternate days. It's considerably more expensive than hydrochlorothiazide and chlorothiazide.

Bendroflumethiazide has been used to suppress breast milk. This further verifies that it shouldn't be used during breast-feeding. It may also worsen a disease called *systemic lupus erythematosis,* if present.

This drug is being tested in the Hypertension in the Elderly Trial in Europe to see if controlling the blood pressure in people age 80 and older causes a substantial reduction in brain attacks among that population.

Hydroflumethiazide

Hydroflumethiazide (Diucardin) comes in 50 mg tablets. The starting dose is one tablet daily, and the maximum dose is 200 mg once daily. In high blood pressure treatment, 25 mg may be sufficient. The kidneys excrete it, so it may accumulate in the presence of kidney disease. In general, it's similar to hydrochlorothiazide in its effects and its side effects.

Methyclorthiazide

Methyclorthiazide (Enduron Tablets, Aquatensen, Methyclorthiazide Tablets) is another variation of hydrochlorothiazide that's ten times as potent as that drug. It's available as 2.5 or 5 mg tablets. It has the same side effects as hydrochlorothiazide.

Polythiazide

Polythiazide (Renese Tablets) is yet another variation on hydrochlorothiazide, but it has 25 times the potency of that medication. It comes in 1, 2, and 4 mg tablets. The lowest dose often lowers blood pressure effectively.

Chlorthalidone

Chlorthalidone (Thalitone, Chlorthalidone Tablets) differs chemically from hydrochlorothiazide, although its blood pressure-lowering activity is about the same. The precautions associated with hydrochlorothiazide pertain to chlorthalidone, which comes as 15 mg tablets. Only half a tablet may be enough to control blood pressure. Its effect tends to last longer.

Indapamide

Indapamide (Lozol) is more like chlorthalidone than hydrochlorothiazide in its structure but has 20 times the potency of that drug. It's available at a dose of 2.5 mg with the usual once or twice daily treatment. However, a sustained release preparation contains 1.5 mg that lasts throughout a 24-hour period with less effect on the potassium than the higher dosage. This dosage is just as effective as 2.0 and 2.5 mg. Indapamide has an advantage over hydrochlorothiazide because it doesn't raise serum cholesterol.

Metolazone

Metolazone (Mykrox, Zaroxolyn) is structurally different from hydrochlorothiazide but acts in much the same way. It's 20 times as potent. The advantage of the preparation of metolazone called Mykrox compared to the preparation called Zaroxolyn is that it's rapidly absorbed and active much earlier than some other diuretics. Mykrox comes in half-milligram tablets. Although it's the same drug, Zaroxolyn is absorbed more slowly and isn't interchangeable with Mykrox. It comes in 2.5, 5, and 10 mg dosages. The precautions for both Mykrox and Zaroxolyn are the same as for hydrochlorothiazide.

Loop diuretics

These drugs are more effective than the thiazide diuretics for ridding the body of salt and water but don't lower the blood pressure as much. When used for high blood pressure treatment, loop diuretics don't raise the cholesterol the way that thiazide diuretics do, a definite advantage; but they're not as effective in reducing disease and death caused by high blood pressure.

Loop diuretics not only reduce the sodium and chloride but the calcium and magnesium as well. They're potent enough to cause a serious fall in the blood sodium if used to excess. They can also cause significant potassium loss. These dangers of loop diuretics make them less useful in the treatment of high blood pressure when compared to thiazide diuretics.

Some of the other problems associated with the loop diuretics include:

✔ Hearing loss or a ringing in the ears

✔ Serum uric acid increase with possible development of gout, a painful swelling of certain joints, especially the big toes

✔ Reactions in those hypersensitive to sulfonamides, which includes several of the drugs for treatment of diabetes, such as diabinase and tolinase and several sulphur-containing antibiotics

✔ When mixed with the following medications, loop diuretics can cause problems:

   • **Anti-inflammatory agents:** Diminishes diuretic activity

   • **Blood thinners:** Tendency to bleed

   • **Digitalis:** Development of irregular heart rhythms

   • **Lithium:** Diarrhea and vomiting

   • **Probenecid:** Diminishes diuretic activity

   • **Propranolol:** An exceptionally slow heart rate

   • **Sulfonylureas:** Low blood sugar

Chemically, loop diuretics are different from one another, unlike the drugs in the thiazide group. Let's take a look at the characteristics of some of the individual loop diuretics.

The loop diuretics are dangerous when the kidneys have failed or sensitivity to the specific drug or to the sulfonamide class of drugs increases. Use during pregnancy and breast-feeding is probably not a good idea but should be discussed with your doctor.

Furosemide

Furosemide (Lasix, Furosemide Tablets, Furosemide Oral Solution) has consistently been the most commonly used member of this group. Although it has a powerful effect on the expulsion of excess salt and water from the body, it can cause excessive salt loss and dehydration because of this, and it shares many of the problems associated with the thiazide diuretics. Among the most important are

- Can't prescribe if kidney failure or hypersensitivity to furosemide or sulfonamide drugs is present
- Must be taken carefully in the presence of severe liver disease
- Not advisable for pregnant or breast-feeding women
- When too much salt and water is lost, dizziness on standing up may result
- Sensitizes skin to the sun
- Associated with increased blood sugar
- Raises the blood uric acid but rarely causes gout
- Advances disease in someone with *systemic lupus erythematosis* (commonly known as *lupus,* a chronic inflammatory disease in which immunological reactions cause abnormalities of blood vessels and connnective tissue)

Furosemide also interacts with many other drugs. Depending on the frequency with which the other drugs are taken, the most important drug interactions include the following:

- Drugs already known to cause damage to hearing, such as aspirin and some antibiotics, may cause even more damage.
- Lithium doesn't clear from the body as much as other drugs and it may cause diarrhea and vomiting.
- Sucralfate, a drug used for treatment of stomach ulcers, may inhibit furosemide activity.

Checking the blood level of sodium, potassium, calcium, and magnesium frequently during the first few months of furosemide treatment is important. Ask your doctor whether your serum sodium and serum potassium are normal after a month of furosemide. If he can't give you an answer, ask to have these tests done every six weeks or so for the first 6 months then occasionally thereafter.

Furosemide comes in 20, 40, and 80 mg tablets. Most patients start by taking the lowest dose, which usually begins to work about an hour after it's taken and lasts for roughly eight hours. If necessary, a second dose can be taken during the day.

Bumetanide

Bumetanide (Bumex, Bumetanide Tablets) is similar in structure and side effects to furosemide but is 40 times more potent. This drug has been associated with severe dehydration and loss of blood electrolytes, such as sodium and potassium.

Bumetanide usually begins to work 30 to 60 minutes after it's taken and lasts for about six hours, but it's usually given once a day in the morning. If a single dose doesn't work long enough, your doctor may prescribe a second dose to be taken later in the day before 6 p.m. to avoid waking up to urinate. Bumetanide is available as half, 1, and 2 mg tablets.

It shares the side effects of the other loop diuretics. Older patients are especially at risk for the severe dehydration that this drug can cause. It hasn't been tested on children under age 18, so it's not recommended for this group.

Ethacrynic acid

Ethacrynic acid (Edecrin Tablets) is also similar in structure to furosemide and is slightly less potent than that drug. It shares the problems of this powerful group of diuretics.

It should probably not be used during pregnancy or breast-feeding.

Ethacrynic acid comes in 25 and 50 mg tablets. For high blood pressure, 25 mg should be taken after a meal. It usually starts to work within 30 minutes and lasts for about eight hours.

Torsemide

Torsemide (Demadex) is the final member of this group. It has three times the potency of furosemide.

The liver does most of the metabolizing of this drug, so torsemide is particularly dangerous in the presence of severe liver disease.

Torsemide is available as 5, 10, 20, and 100 mg tablets. It can be taken any time in relation to a meal. It usually begins to work an hour after it's taken and continues for about 8 hours. For high blood pressure patients, the lowest dose is usually given and not changed until 4 to 6 weeks have passed. Ten milligrams is usually the maximum dose given for the treatment of high blood pressure.

Potassium-sparing diuretics

These drugs have little effect on salt and water or lowering blood pressure, but used in combination with other diuretics, they conserve the body's potassium. They're often manufactured together with a diuretic to form a combination.

Not only do these drugs conserve potassium, but they also decrease the loss of calcium and magnesium that's associated with the other diuretics.

Their ability to conserve potassium is the source of their greatest danger, which is an abnormal elevation of the blood-potassium level, so they should never be used when the potassium is already high. People with diseases such as kidney failure are at a particularly high risk for this complication.

Amiloride

Amiloride (Midamor Tablets, Amiloride HCl Tablets) is used only with another diuretic to reverse the tendency of the other diuretic to excrete potassium in the urine. So, along with potassium, it also conserves magnesium.

This drug comes in a 5 mg tablet, the usual dose. It starts to act two hours after it's taken and continues its activity for 24 hours.

Amiloride is eliminated by the kidneys and by the liver to about the same extent. Amiloride in the presence of kidney failure or liver disease is dangerous because it can accumulate and become toxic.

Amiloride may also cause excessive potassium retention so potassium levels in the blood must be monitored. Muscle weakness, swelling of the abdomen, and diarrhea are symptomatic of excessive potassium retention. Patients who have diabetes mellitus (discussed in Chapter 4) are especially sensitive to the potassium-sparing effect of amiloride, even when they don't have kidney disease. Using salt substitutes can probably put someone who's taking amiloride at greater risk because salt substitutes contain potassium chloride instead of sodium chloride.

Amiloride isn't recommended during pregnancy or breast-feeding. It can decrease the excretion of lithium in the urine leading to lithium toxicity.

Triamterene

Triamterene (Dyrenium) differs in structure from amiloride and has only a tenth of the potency of that drug. It accomplishes the same task of conserving potassium in the patient getting another diuretic that causes potassium loss.

Triamterene comes as 50 and 100 mg tablets. It usually starts to act two to four hours after it's taken, and its action lasts for up to nine hours. As a result, it usually must be taken twice a day, which is a disadvantage. It's taken after meals to avoid stomach upset.

It has to be monitored just like amiloride with frequent tests of blood potassium, especially in people with diabetes and the elderly, who are more likely to have high blood potassium levels. It's not recommended during pregnancy and breast-feeding.

Because it leaves the body in the urine, it accumulates when kidney failure is present and shouldn't be taken in this situation or when liver disease exists.

Antagonist of aldosterone: spironolactone

Spironolactone (Aldactone) is not a diuretic in the sense that it directly causes loss of salt and potassium in the urine. It blocks the action of the steroid hormone aldosterone (see Chapter 6). Because aldosterone causes salt and water retention, spironolactone causes salt and water loss only if aldosterone is present. As salt is lost, potassium is conserved, so spironolactone is a potassium-sparing drug. It must be used carefully when potassium is already elevated or a drug that tends to raise potassium is being used. All the information about the danger of high potassium for amiloride and triamterene (discussed in the "Amiloride" and "Triamterene" sections previously) applies to spironolactone.

The drug comes in 25, 50, and 100 mg tablets. It usually starts to act after only one to two days and continues to increase salt and urine output for two to three days. For high blood pressure, 50 mg a day is usually prescribed with a diuretic that causes potassium loss. Your doctor may be willing to reduce the dose to 25 mg with a good result.

Spironolactone has a number of side effects because of its structure. It can cause breast enlargement in men and women, loss of potency, decreased interest in sex, increased hairiness, deepening of the voice, and menstrual irregularities. It can also cause irritation and bleeding in the stomach. Finally, it may cause sleepiness, confusion, and headache.

Diuretic combinations

If a thiazide diuretic is prescribed at the recommended low dosage, the possibility of excessive potassium loss is small, especially when the person eats a good diet, but it does occur. At higher doses, potassium loss is more likely. Because of the thiazide diuretics' tendency to cause potassium loss, drug companies have created a number of diuretic combinations. You may already be taking one or another of the combinations (listed here by their brand names) that follow:

- **Amiloride HCl and HCTZ Tablets:** 5 mg amiloride plus 50 mg hydrochlorothiazide
- **Amiloride Hydrochloride and Hydrochlorothiazide Tablets:** 5 mg amiloride plus 50 mg hydrochlorothiazide
- **Dyazide:** 37.5 mg triamterene and 25 mg hydrochlorothiazide

- **Maxide:** 75 mg Triamterene and 50 mg hydrochlorothiazide

- **Maxide-25:** 37.5 mg Triamterene and 25 mg hydrochlorothiazide

- **Moduretic:** 5 mg amiloride plus 50 mg hydrochlorothiazide

- **Triamterene and Hydrochlorothiazide Capsules and Tablets:** 37.5 mg triamterene and 25 mg hydrochlorothiazide

- **Triamterene and Hydrochlorothiazide Tablets:** 75 mg triamterene and 25 mg hydrochlorothiazide

- **Triamterene/HCTZ Capsules:** 50 mg triamterene and 25 mg hydrochlorothiazide

- **Triamterene/HCTZ Capsules and Tablets:** 37.5 mg triamterene and 25 mg hydrochlorothiazide

- **Triamterene/HCTZ Tablets:** 75 mg triamterene and 50 mg hydrochlorothiazide

- **Spironolactone and Hydrochlorothiazide Tablets:** 25 mg spironolactone and 25 mg hydrochlorothiazide

As you can see, numerous choices of tablets and capsules are available in numerous amounts. Make sure that you're getting the combination that your doctor wants you to have.

Drugs That Act on the Nervous System

The part of the nervous system that's responsible for increased constriction of the arteries, thus raising blood pressure, is *the sympathetic nervous system*. In 1940, researchers discovered that cutting the nerves of the sympathetic nervous system in the chest and abdomen caused a persistent fall in blood pressure. Since then, scientists have looked for chemical agents that could block the sympathetic nervous system, and they have come up with quite a bundle. They're broken down into groups by the way they affect the nervous system. I list each medication together with the others that lower blood pressure in the same way, but don't worry, I will explain each group in English terms.

Methyldopa

Methyldopa (Aldomet, Methyldopa Tablets), a drug that acts within the brain to prevent the release of neurotransmitters so they never get to the receptors, has been an effective drug in the past and is still used by many physicians. It isn't usually the first drug of choice for high blood pressure because of the following rare but serious side effects:

Blocking the sympathetic nervous system

The sympathetic nervous system uses hormones called *epinephrine* and *norepinehrine* to act as chemical messengers called *neurotransmitters* along the nerves. When the brain wants action, such as blood vessel constriction, it sends out neurotransmitters that are found in storage vesicles. These neurotransmitters make the jump from the end of one nerve to the beginning of another nerve. Receptors located at the beginning of nerves take up the neurotransmitter, so the signal can proceed down the nerve. Various drugs lower blood pressure by affecting nerve transmission in the brain or outside the brain.

✔ **Anemia:** Iron-deficient blood that causes red blood cell count to fall

✔ **Liver damage:** With fever and abnormal liver blood tests

Because of these side effects, patients should have their blood count checked and liver tests done before the drug is started and again every few months for the first year. If anemia and/or liver damage is discovered, stop taking the drug and these side effects usually disappear.

Other side effects include

✔ **Decreased sex drive:** Some patients complain of decreased sexual interest.

✔ **Dry mouth:** A dry mouth may result from decreased saliva production.

✔ **Elevated levels of prolactin:** An elevated level of the brain hormone prolactin, which can cause an increase in breast size and formation of liquid in the breasts.

✔ **Sleepiness:** When Methyldopa is first prescribed, driving and running other complicated machinery should be done cautiously.

The drug has been found safe for pregnant women and is often the first choice for pregnant women with high blood pressure. It's found in breast milk, however, so it's not the best choice for a nursing mother.

Methyldopa comes in 125, 250, and 500 mg tablets. It usually begins to work two hours after it's taken and its effect lasts for about eight hours. It's usually given at a dose of 250 mg two or three times a day and raised or lowered every few days until blood pressure control is achieved. The maximum dose is four 500 mg tablets a day. Methyldopa is eliminated from the body through the kidneys for the most part, so patients who have reduced kidney function require lower doses.

A combination of methyldopa and other drugs for high blood pressure, especially the thiazide diuretics, can be very effective. The various combinations of methyldopa and other drugs for high blood pressure include:

- **Aldoclor:** A combination of methyldopa and chlorothiazide has 250 mg of each drug.

- **Aldoril:** A combination of methyldopa and hydrochlorothiazide comes in four different strengths:

  - **Aldoril-15:** 250 mg methyldopa and 15 mg hydrochlorothiazide
  - **Aldoril-25:** 250 mg methyldopa and 25 mg hyrdrochlorothiazide
  - **Aldoril-D30:** 500 mg methyldopa and 30 mg hydrochlorothiazide
  - **Aldoril D50:** 500 mg methyldopa and 50 mg hydrochlorothiazide

- **Methyldopa and Hydrochlorothiazide Tablets:** 250 mg methyldopa and 15 mg hydrochlorothiazide; or 250 mg methyldopa and 25 mg hydrochlorothiazide

Clonidine, Guanabenz, and Guanfacine

Clonidine (Catapres, Clonidine Hydrochloride Tablets, Clonidine HCl Tablets), guanabenz (Wytensin, Guanabenz Acetate Tablets) and guanfacine (Tenex, Guanfacine Tablets, Guanfacine Hydrochloride Tablets) are similar drugs that lower blood pressure by reducing levels of the chemical messenger norepinephrine that increases blood pressure. They reduce the output of blood from the heart and increase the size of arteries. Because of the sedation that they bring on (and the better characteristics of other drugs), they aren't the drug of choice for treating high blood pressure.

- **Clonidine** comes in 0.1, 0.2, and 0.3 mg strengths. It's usually prescribed as a starting dose of 0.1 mg twice daily and changed on a weekly basis depending on the blood pressure. The maximum dose is usually 0.6 mg although some doctors use more. It usually begins to act within an hour and lasts for roughly 12 hours

  Clonidine is also marketed as a patch that can be applied to the skin. It's called Catapres-TTS, Catapres transdermal system. The patch contains 0.1, 0.2, or 0.3 mg. Each patch lasts a week as long as it doesn't fall off.

- **Guanabenz** comes as 4 and 8 mg tablets. It's usually started at 4 mg twice daily and increased to 8 mg twice daily. The maximum dose is 32 mg. It usually begins to act in 60 minutes and lasts about 12 hours. The dose may be changed every two weeks until the blood pressure is under control.

✔ **Guanfacine** comes in 1 or 2 mg tablets. It's usually started at 1 mg at bedtime. It begins to work in about two hours and lasts for roughly 24 hours. It can be changed every three to four weeks up to a maximum dose of 3 mg daily.

These three drugs have similar side effects including

✔ **Sleepiness:** Best taken before bedtime; dosage increases are made at bedtime.

✔ **Dry mouth:** May worsen to dry eyes and dryness of the nose.

✔ **Disturbing dreams:** Sometimes clonidine, guanabenz, or guanfacine may cause vivid dreams or nightmares and depression.

If these drugs are discontinued, especially at higher doses, it must be done gradually because of withdrawal symptoms, such as headache and shakiness as well as a rise in arterial blood pressure above the original blood pressure for which the drug was started. For this reason, if your doctor recommends that you quit taking the drug before surgery, he'll probably substitute another drug well in advance. Or he may not stop this drug at all but be sure that you get the drug on the morning of your surgery.

These drugs are usually given with a diuretic, and several preparations that combine the two are available including the following:

✔ **Combipres:** 0.1, 0.2, or 0.3 mg Clonidine with 15 mg chlorthalidone

✔ **Clorpres:** This is the same as Combipres, but from another company.

Beta-adrenergic receptor blockers

Beta-adrenergic receptor blockers, generally known as beta blockers, are the most important group of drugs that affect the sympathetic nervous system and are second only to the thiazide diuretics in their effectiveness.

So many of them are available that it seems as though each drug manufacturer has its own version. Given all the choices, how do you know which beta blocker is best for you? Although they differ in certain respects, they all seem to have about the same effect on the blood pressure. In this respect, they're only slightly less effective than the diuretics. They're added when the thiazide diuretics don't completely control the blood pressure.

Beta blockers aren't the drug of choice for high blood pressure unless the patient has a history of chest pain or heart attack. Beta blockers reduce the forcefulness of the heart while they reduce the secretion of renin and the production of angiotensin II (see Chapter 6). They seem to protect those with atherosclerotic heart disease (see Chapter 5) against pain and further disease.

Two different beta-adrenergic receptors blockers interrupt the sympathetic nervous system's activity: beta 1 and beta 2. Beta-1 blockers block against beta-1 receptors while beta-2 blockers block against beta-2 receptors. As the dose of the beta blocker rises, their specificity declines, and the same beta blocker blocks both receptors.

Beta blockers are especially useful for people with diseased blood vessels in the heart. This is particularly true of the beta-2 blockers, such as propranolol and timolol, that don't attach selectively to the nerves in the heart. Studies have shown that these drugs were associated with a reduction in death rates while the other beta-1 blockers were not. Choosing between propranolol and timolol comes down to cost. Twice-daily propranolol is much less expensive than twice-daily timolol. Make sure the nonbrand named drug is used. If you want to make life a little easier (but more expensive), you can choose Inderal LA for once-a-day dosing.

Of all the beta blockers, based on the scientific evidence, propranolol is probably the best choice.

Beta blockers are associated with a number of side effects. The important ones are

- **Fatigue:** This may result from the decrease in blood flow to the brain when the blood pressure is lowered.
- **Slows heart rate:** Part of the tendency toward fatigue.
- **Blocks heart:** When the electrical conduction system of the heart is diseased, beta blockers can be harmful.
- **Intolerance to exercise:** Not a good choice for the strenuous exerciser.
- **Aggravates asthma:** They can make asthma worse.
- **Lowers blood HDL:** Some of the beta blockers lower the blood HDL, the good cholesterol.
- **Toxicity:** In the presence of kidney failure or liver disease, beta blockers can accumulate because they're eliminated by the kidneys, the liver, or both.
- **Can increase blood pressure if stopped:** If the drugs are suddenly stopped, the blood pressure may rebound up higher than the pre-treatment level. They should be lowered gradually over a couple of weeks.
- **Lowered blood sugar:** Diabetics who take these drugs may not respond properly to low blood sugar levels because the hormones that raise the blood sugar are dependent on the nerves that are blocked by beta blockers.

✓ **Heart attack:** Beta blockers have to be discontinued slowly to avoid precipitating heart pain and a heart attack.

✓ **Retards fetal growth:** They should not be used during pregnancy because the growth of the fetus may be retarded.

Beta blockers were thought to be less effective for the elderly, but this is no longer considered the case. They're less practical for the African American diabetic population, however. Beta blockers aren't as effective among the African American population as they are in other people. The exception is labetalol, a drug that's a combined beta and alpha blocker.

The characteristics of the various beta blockers, which can be spotted since their scientific names end in "lol" are as follows:

✓ **Acebutolol** (Sectral, Acebutolol Capsules, Acebutolol Hydrochloride Capsules) comes in 200 or 400 mg capsules. It's usually prescribed for once daily starting at 200 mg up to a maximum of 1200 mg. The liver eliminates acebutolol more than the kidney.

✓ **Atenolol** (Tenormin, Atenolol Tablets) is available in 25, 50, or 100 mg tablets. The starting dose is usually 25 mg once a day up to a maximum of 200 mg once a day.

Atenolol also comes in combination form as Tenoretic 50, which is 50 mg of atenolol and 25 mg of the diuretic, chlorthalidone; and Tenoretic 100, which is 100 mg of atenolol and 25 mg of chlorthalidone. Atenolol and Chlorthalidone Tablets are the same two combinations by another drug company. Atenolol in any form is eliminated by the kidney.

✓ **Bisoprolol** (Zebeta) is supplied as 5 and 10 mg tablets. For high blood pressure, the starting dose is usually 5 mg, and some may do well with half that dose. The maximum dose is 20 mg. The characteristics of bisoprolol are similar to all other members of this group. Bisoprolol is eliminated by both the kidneys and the liver so disease of either organ will increase blood levels of the drug.

✓ **Carteolol** (Cartrol Filmtab Tablets) is sold as a 2.5 or a 5 mg tablet. 2.5 mg is usually taken once a day up to a maximum of 10 mg once daily. This drug is eliminated more by the kidney than the liver.

✓ **Carvedilol** (Coreg) comes as 3.125, 6.25, 12.5, and 25 mg tablets. The starting dose is usually 6.25 mg twice daily up to a maximum of 50 mg divided into two doses. The liver breaks down carvedilol. People with liver disease may accumulate this drug in their bloodstream.

✓ **Labetalol** (Normodyne, Trandate, Labetalol HCl Tablets) comes as 100, 200, and 300 mg tablets. It differs from most of the other beta blockers because of its effect on other receptors called *alpha receptors.* This often causes dizziness, and the drug has been associated with fever and liver abnormalities. The dose is usually 100 mg twice daily up to 1200 mg divided into two doses. The liver is the major organ of elimination.

✔ **Metoprolol** (Lopressor, Metoprolol Tartrate Tablets) are made in 50 mg and 100 mg strengths. The usual dose is 50 mg once a day up to a maximum of 200 mg once a day.

A slow-release form of the this drug called Toprol XL is usually prescribed for once a day. It comes in 50, 100, and 200 mg tablets. Elimination of both metoprolol and Toprol XL is by the liver.

✔ **Nadolol** (Nadolol Tablets) comes in 20, 40, and 80 mg tablets. The starting dose is usually 20 mg once daily up to 160 mg once daily. The kidney is the main site of elimination.

Nadolol also comes in combination with a thiazide diuretic, bendroflumethiazide (discussed earlier in this chapter in the "Thiazide and thiazidelike diuretic group" section) that's called Corzide. The tablets are either 40 mg of nadolol with 5 mg of bendroflumethiazide or 80 mg of nadolol with 5 mg of bendroflumethiazide.

✔ **Penbutolol** (Levatol) comes as a 20 mg tablet. The dose is usually 20 mg once a day up to 80 mg once a day. The kidneys eliminate penbutolol more than the liver.

✔ **Pindolol** (Pindolol Tablets) is made in 5 and 10 mg strengths. The dose is usually 5 mg twice daily up to a maximum of 60 mg divided into two doses. The liver eliminates more of this drug than the kidneys.

✔ **Propranolol** (Inderal Tablets, Propranolol Hydrochloride Oral Solution, Propranolol Hydrochloride Tablets) comes in 10, 20, 40, 60, and 80 mg strengths. The initial prescription is usually for 20 mg twice daily up to 320 mg divided into two doses. This was the earliest of the beta blockers, and therefore doctors have the most experience with it. It's eliminated by the liver.

Propranolol also comes in a long-acting form called Inderal LA, which is made in 60, 80, 120, or 160 mg strengths. This allows for once-a-day dosing. It's also made in combination with hydrochlorothiazide called Inderide or Propranolol Hydrochloride, and Hydrochlorothiazide Tablets come in two different strengths, 40 and 80 mg of propranolol plus 25 mg hydrochlorothiazide. Finally, a long-acting preparation of Inderide called Inderide LA contains 80, 120, or 160 mg of propranolol plus 50 mg hydrochlorothiazide and can be taken once a day.

✔ **Timolol** (Blocadren, Timolol Maleate Tablets) comes as 5, 10, or 20 mg tablets. The dose is usually 5 mg twice daily up to 40 mg divided into two doses. Timolol is eliminated by the liver more than the kidneys.

Timolol is also manufactured in combination with hydrochlorothiazide as Timolide consisting of 10 mg of timolol and 25 mg of the diuretic. It also comes in solutions for the eye that lower elevated pressure in the eye.

Alpha-1 adrenergic receptor antagonists

Alpha-1 adrenergic receptor antagonists block another group of sympathetic nerve receptors, some of which are alpha 1 and some alpha 2. Only the alpha-1 blockers are used clinically.

Alpha-1 drugs act through different nerve receptors to increase the size of arteries. They can be associated with dizziness on standing. They lower the bad fats, triglycerides and LDL cholesterol and raise the good fat, HDL cholesterol. The changes are small, however.

Some unwanted side effects of these drugs include

- Increased occurrence of heart failure

- *First-dose phenomenon* where the blood pressure drops down low after the first dose or when the drug is rapidly increased. This is especially true for patients already on a diuretic or a beta blocker. Avoiding driving or difficult tasks is advisable for the first 24 hours after the first dose, which is best given at bedtime. This goes away after the first few doses.

Their tendency to cause heart failure means taking them alone isn't recommended, but rather they should be combined with a diuretic. They also may lose their potency after a while when the body gets used to them.

The various drugs in this group include the following:

- **Doxazocin** (Cardura) is made in 1, 2, 4, and 8 mg tablets with a starting dose of 1 mg at bedtime. This can go up to 16 mg once a day. It has been used in benign prostatic hypertrophy as well as high blood pressure. It's not a good choice for a pregnant or nursing woman. Dizziness and fatigue occur in many of the patients who take it. It's eliminated by the liver.

- **Prazosin** (Minipress, Prazosin HCl Capsules, Prazosin Hydrochloride Capsules, Prazosin HCl Capsules) comes as 1, 2, and 5 mg tablets. It's usually given at a starting dose of 1 mg at bedtime up to 20 mg in two or three divided doses. Prazosin isn't recommended for women who are pregnant or breast-feeding.

  Prazosin is also produced as Minizide, a combination of 1, 2, or 5 mg of prazosin with 0.5 mg Polythiazide, a thiazide diruetic. The liver breaks it down, and the drug is eliminated in the feces.

- **Terazosin** (Hytrin, Terazosin Capsules, Terazosin Hydrochloride Capsules, Terazosin Tablets) is produced in 1, 2, 5, and 10 mg strengths. The initial dose is 1 mg at bedtime rising to 20 mg divided into 2 doses if necessary. It also may reduce the size of the prostate gland in men. The liver eliminates terazosin.

These drugs were used more in the past than in the present because their tendency to cause side effects has made them less popular. It's preferable to use them with a thiazide diuretic.

Vasodilators

Vasodilators are drugs that relax the muscles in the arteries, making them larger and reducing blood pressure. How this occurs is unclear. If these drugs are given alone, the heart speeds up as the blood pressure falls and patients suffer from headaches, the feeling of a rapid heart beat, and retention of water. Therefore, they're usually given with diuretics to get rid of water and beta blockers to slow the heart. Doctors use two vasodilators, hydralazine and minoxidil, usually for the most difficult cases because of their side effects. I describe each drug in the following sections.

Hydralazine

Hydralazine (Apresoline, Hydralazine HCl Tablets) was one of the earliest drugs used for high blood pressure. It wasn't prescribed often at first because of the side effects of rapid heart beat and loss of effectiveness after taking it for a while. The loss of effectiveness results from the body compensating for the opening wide of the blood vessels by increasing heart rate and retaining water. When this was understood, other drugs could be given to counteract this compensation, and hydralazine was restored to effectiveness.

Hydralazine is available in 25 and 50 mg strengths. It's usually administered twice daily because its action lasts about 12 hours. The maximum dose is 200 mg divided into two doses. The drug is broken down mostly in the liver. About half the population breaks down the drug rapidly (they're called *fast acetylators*) while the other half breaks it down more slowly *(slow acetylators)*. Once the drug is broken down in the liver, it's no longer active, so the fast acetylators need more of the drug.

Hydralazine is also available in combination form as Hydra-Zide Capsules. This is a combination of hydralazine and hydrochlorothiazide in the following proportions: 25 mg hydralazine and 25 mg hydrochlorothiazide, 50 mg hydralazine and 50 mg hydrochlorothiazide, 100 mg hydralazine and 50 mg hydrochlorothiazide.

Anyone with liver disease must take this drug with care. This is true for people with kidney disease as well because the drug is eliminated by the kidneys.

Hydralazine's side effects include headaches, nausea, excess reduction in blood pressure, feeling of a rapid heartbeat, dizziness, and heart pain if there is coronary artery disease. Interestingly, although hydralazine expands some arteries of the heart, it doesn't expand certain other arteries in the heart. The result is that blood is "stolen" from one area to another. The area that loses blood may develop pain.

Hydralazine also causes retention of water and can result in heart failure, so it's usually given with both a diuretic and a beta blocker.

Hydralazine also causes the occurrence of an allergic reaction against the body's own tissues called the *lupus syndrome.* This begins only after at least six months of treatment and is more frequent as the dose goes higher. Slow acetylators get this condition more often than fast acetylators. The symptoms consist of fever, rash, itching, pain in the joints and actual swelling, redness and heat in the joints. After the drug is stopped, the condition usually subsides.

Hydralazine is rarely used alone or in elderly patients because of the side effects. It has been prescribed for pregnant women and has been useful for severe high blood pressure during pregnancy. However, it shouldn't be prescribed to a nursing mother.

Minoxidil

Minoxidil (Loniten, Minoxidil Tablets) was first discovered in 1965 and was found to control the most severe and resistant cases of high blood pressure. Its action is to relax *smooth muscle,* the muscle that's found in the walls of arteries. Minoxidil is most useful for severe high blood pressure that doesn't respond to other agents. It's always administered with a diuretic and a beta blocker to reverse the undesirable side effects listed later in this section.

Minoxidil is available in 2.5 and 10 mg tablets. The starting dose may be as little as 1.25 mg once daily up to a maximum of 40 mg once daily. It begins to work about 30 minutes after it's taken. The drug is broken down in the liver, but it's also eliminated by the kidneys, so disease of either of these organs causes minoxidil to accumulate in the body.

Minoxidil has been used in children, but it's not recommended for pregnant women or women who are breast-feeding. The following side effects, however, complicate the use of this powerful drug:

✔ Salt and water are retained because the pressure in the kidney's nephrons (see Chapter 6) is reduced. Giving a diuretic along with the minoxidil reverses this.

✔ The heart rate increases along with the strength of heart contractions. If coronary artery disease already exists, heart pain can result from the increased work of the heart. A beta-blocking drug can control this side effect. If the heart has been close to failure, this drug may worsen the problem so that heart failure occurs.

> ✔ Increased hair growth on the face, back, arms, and legs develops in all patients on minoxidil for several months or more. This is a problem for women especially. Minoxidil is now used commercially in the form of Rogaine for treatment of baldness.

Calcium Channel Blocking Agents

Calcium channel blocking agents (also known as calcium channel blockers) take advantage of the fact that in order for a muscle in an artery to contract to make the artery smaller, calcium has to move into the muscle cell. These agents block that movement, and the muscle relaxes, resulting in larger arteries and lower blood pressure.

As arteries widen and peripheral resistance declines, the body responds by increasing the heart rate. This isn't true of all calcium channel blocking agents, however. Certain calcium channel blocking agents, particularly verapamil, nifedipine, and diltiazem (see more on these drugs later in this section), slow the heart, so the heart rate doesn't increase when these are used.

Calcium channel blockers aren't the first or second drug of choice for blood pressure treatment among people with enlarged hearts or when heart failure is present. Calcium channel blockers also shouldn't be the first or second choice of treatment for high blood pressure after a heart attack. They decrease muscle contraction, an undesirable effect when the heart is already failing or weakened by a heart attack.

When heart disease doesn't already exist, calcium channel blockers can lower blood pressure as effectively as beta blockers. When a heart attack has occurred, calcium channel blockers don't improve survival the way that beta blockers do.

These drugs have several side effects, but these side effects rarely cause the patient to stop taking the drug. The main side effects are headache, flushing in the face, dizziness, and swelling of the legs. To overcome these side effects, sustained-release preparations have been developed.

Another side effect that may make the patient uncomfortable is irritation of the *esophagus* (the passageway from the mouth to the stomach) and the stomach. This occurs because these agents slow food passage from the stomach to the intestine. Constipation is also common.

Calcium channel blockers are effective in most patients when the preceding problems are taken into account. They work especially well in low renin high blood pressure, the situation most often found among the elderly and African Americans. Of course, heart failure and heart attacks are most often found in the elderly as well, so this is a consideration.

Interactions with other drugs are important. The metabolism of digoxin, an important drug for the heart, is blocked, so digoxin can accumulate to toxic levels, resulting in severe abnormal heart rhythms.

These agents are safe in the presence of diabetes, asthma, kidney abnormalities, and when blood fats are abnormal. So calcium channel blockers can be useful, even though they're not the first choice for treating high blood pressure.

A number of calcium channel blockers are available and are classified by their chemical structure. One group, that does not have the same underlying chemical structure, consists of verapamil and diltiazem. The second group, all connected by having a similar chemical structure, consist of amlodipine, felodipine, asradipine, nicardipine, nifedipine and nisoldipine, all of which end in "pine." Some of their important features are as follows:

- ✔ **Verapamil** (Isoptin, Calan, Verelan, Covera, Verapamil HCl Tablets, Verapamil Hydrochloride Tablets) is available in tablets containing 40, 80, and 120 mg of the drug. The dose is usually 80 mg three times a day up to 360 mg divided into three doses. Most of the drug is excreted into the urine but about 20 percent leaves in the feces. When liver or kidney disease is present, the drug may accumulate.

  Long-acting preparations of verapamil are available:

  - **Calan SR** containing 120, 180, or 240 mg may be taken once a day with food.

  - **Covera-HS** is available as 180 and 240 mg tablets given at bedtime.

  - **Isoptin SR** is identical to Calan SR.

  - **Verelan** is a sustained-release capsule available in strengths of 120, 180, 240, and 360 mg and may be taken once in the morning.

  - **Verelan PM** is a capsule containing either 100, 200, or 300 mg of verapamil and is taken at bedtime.

  - **Verapamil Hydrochloride Extended-release Capsules and Tablets** are similar to Calan SR.

- ✔ **Diltiazem** (Cardizem CD Capsules, Tiazac, Diltiazem Extended Release Capsules, Diltiazem Hydrochloride Extended Release Capsules, Diltiazem Hydrochloride Tablets) is usually sold in the extended release form for once-a-day dosing. It comes in 120, 180, 240, 300, and 360 mg capsules and tablets. The starting dose is usually 180 mg daily up to 360 mg once daily maximum. The liver processes diltiazem, so toxicity is likely to occur in the presence of liver disease. However, decreased kidney function doesn't seem to affect it. The side effects of diltiazem are just like those of verapamil, but it's more likely to cause constipation and heart failure.

- ✔ **Amlodipine** (Lotrel, Norvasc) is manufactured as 2.5, 5, and 10 mg tablets. It's usually prescribed in the beginning at the 5 mg level once daily going up to a maximum of 10 mg once a day. Elderly people usually start at 2.5 mg. It's broken down in the liver, and the breakdown products are eliminated in the urine. Liver disease causes amlodipine to accumulate, but kidney disease doesn't affect the dosing. A small number of men complain of impotency with this drug. Few patients have to stop it because of side effects, so these aren't severe. Amlodipine doesn't often interact with other drugs. Amlodipine isn't recommended during pregnancy or when breast-feeding.

✔ **Felodipine** (Plendil) comes as an extended-release tablet in 2.5, 5, and 10 mg strengths. The starting dose is usually 5 mg, and the maximum is 10 mg once a day. It's taken without food or with a light meal and swallowed whole. The elimination and side effects of amlodipine apply to felodipine as do the maternal and breast-feeding precautions. Felodipine also comes in combination with enalapril (see more on this later in the "Angiotensin-converting enzyme inhibitors" section) in a product called Lexxel, which is manufactured as 5 mg of enalapril and 2.5 or 5 mg of felodipine.

✔ **Nicardipine** (Cardene, Nicardipine Capsules, Nicardipine Hydrochloride) comes as 20 and 30 mg capsules. The starting dose is usually 20 mg three times daily and the maximum dose is 120 mg divided in three doses. This three-times-a-day dosing is a definite disadvantage when compared to the others of this group. It shares all the characteristics of amlodipine.

✔ **Nifedipine** (Adalat Capsules, Procardia Capsules) is available as 10 or 20 mg capsules. The dose is usually 10 mg three times daily up to 120 mg divided into three doses.

Because of the inconvenience of three daily doses, extended-release formulations called Adalat CC Extended Release Tablets, Procardia XL Extended Release Tablets, and Nifedipine Extended-release Tablets are available. These come in strengths of 30, 60 and 90 mg. The description of the side effects of amlodipine apply to nifedipine.

✔ **Nisoldipine** (Sular) is an extended-release tablet available in strengths of 10, 20, 30, and 40 mg. The starting dose is usually 20 mg once a day up to a maximum of 60 mg once a day. This drug shouldn't be taken with a high-fat meal, which leads to excessive release and a high concentration. Otherwise, the description of nisoldipine doesn't differ from amlodipine.

Given all the choices, which of these is the best for you? Remember, first of all, that a calcium channel blocker isn't the drug of choice for treating high blood pressure. If a combination of a diuretic and a beta blocker aren't sufficient, these drugs may be considered. The second group of drugs from amlodipine on down are slightly more effective than diltiazem and verapamil, although the latter two drugs have fewer side effects. Little difference exists among the second group, so it's reasonable to choose the least expensive extended-release tablet, which would be Nifedipine Extended-release Tablets. Naturally, you don't get to make the decision, but you can influence your doctor if you come prepared with the information in this chapter.

Angiotensin-Converting Enzyme Inhibitors

Angiotensin-converting enzyme (ACE) *inhibitors* affect the activity of the renin-angiotensin-aldosterone system (see Chapter 6). Angiotensin-converting enzyme converts a hormone called angiotensin I to angiotensin II. Angiotensin II raises blood pressure two ways: It causes direct contraction of arteries, and it causes the adrenal gland to release aldosterone (see Chapter 4), which, in turn, causes salt and water retention. The ACE inhibitors block the angiotensin-converting enzyme so that angiotensin II isn't made. ACE inhibitors can make thiazide diuretics more effective by blocking the tendency of the body to make more aldosterone as water and salt are lost.

While it prevents the increase in blood pressure, the ACE inhibitor also leads to a fall in blood pressure because angiotensin II also breaks down *bradykinen,* a hormone that causes widening of blood vessels. In the absence of angiotensin II, *bradykinen* levels are increased.

This class of drugs is especially important for people with heart failure, kidney disease, diabetes, and other kidney problems. More than any other drug for high blood pressure, ACE inhibitors slow the progression of these diseases, so they're especially useful when these conditions are present.

One advantage of the ACE inhibitors is that they don't cause changes in blood fats, blood sugar, and uric acid, or a fall in potassium. Another major advantage of the ACE inhibitors is the low number of side effects. Potential side effects include

- By blocking aldosterone production, they may lead to elevations in serum potassium levels, especially in patients with heart failure or reduced kidney function.

- They can lead to abnormally low blood pressure if the patient has decreased blood volume to begin with as, for example, after treatment with a diuretic.

- Most of them cause a dry cough in 20 percent of the patients who receive the drug, which can be very annoying.

   Rare side effects include a rash, loss of taste, and reduction of white blood cells.

A very rare but potentially fatal complication is *angioneurotic edema,* which causes the throat to swell severely and breathing is troubled. These drugs should be stopped immediately if such signs and symptoms develop.

An ACE inhibitor paired with a potassium-sparing diuretic or spironolactone can be dangerous because both cause increase blood potassium.

ACE inhibitors should absolutely not be used during pregnancy or in a young woman who plans to become pregnant soon because they've been known to damage the growing fetus. Likewise, they shouldn't be used during breast-feeding to avoid damage to the nursing infant.

These drugs aren't as effective among African Americans unless given with a diuretic, probably because their high blood pressure isn't driven by angiotensin II. The elderly respond just like younger people.

When ACE inhibitors are compared with diuretics, beta blockers, and calcium channel blockers, they don't lower blood pressure as effectively as these other drugs. When compared in terms of decreasing sickness and death, ACE inhibitors aren't as effective as diuretics or beta blockers but better than calcium channel blockers.

Numerous ACE inhibitors are available with some variation in their breakdown. They can be recognized by the fact that their names end in "pril". Their characteristics are as follows:

- **Benazepril** (Lotensin), available as 5, 10, 20, and 40 mg tablets, is usually prescribed initially at a dose of 10 mg daily rising to 40 mg daily if needed or it can be divided into two doses. Patients who are already receiving a diuretic are at risk for very low blood pressure when benazepril is started. Stopping the diuretic for several days first is recommended, and then adding it back if the ACE inhibitor doesn't control the blood pressure. Alternately, the starting dose of benazepril can be 5 mg. Because the kidneys eliminate this drug in part, patients with severe kidney function loss need to take reduced doses.

  Benazepril is also available in combination with hydrochlorothiazide as Lotensin HCT. The proportions are benazepril 5 mg, hydrochlorothiazide 6.25 mg, 10 mg/12.5 mg, 20 mg/12.5 mg, and 20 mg/25 mg. Benazepril is also packaged with the calcium channel blocker amlodipine as Lotrel. The proportions are 2.5 mg amlodipine and 10 mg benazepril, 5 mg/10 mg, and 5 mg/20 mg.

- **Captopril** (Capoten, Captopril Tablets) was the first of the ACE inhibitors. It comes in 12.5, 25, 50 and 100 mg strengths. It's usually started at 25 mg twice daily and increased up to 150 mg daily in two or three doses. Food decreases the uptake of this drug. It should be taken an hour before meals. Most of the drug is eliminated in the urine, so people with decreased kidney function will take less. Captopril seems to cause skin rashes and problems with taste more often than the other ACE inhibitors. The same precaution for a patient already on a diuretic mentioned for benazepril applies to captopril and all the other ACE inhibitors.

  Captopril is also sold together with hydrochlorothiazide as Captopril and Hydrochlorothiazide Tablets. The proportions are captopril 25 mg, hydrochlorothiazide 15 mg, 50 mg/15 mg, 25 mg/25 mg, and 50 mg/25 mg.

✔ **Enalapril** (Vasotec) comes in 2.5, 5, 10, and 20 mg tablets. The usual dose is 5 mg once a day rising to 40 mg once a day or divided into two doses. The kidneys eliminate it, so less is taken in the presence of diminished kidney function.

Vaseretic is a combination of enalapril and hydrochlorothiazide in the following proportions: 5 mg/12.5 mg and 10 mg/25 mg. Lexxel has been described under "Felodipine" earlier in this chapter with which enalapril is combined to make this drug.

✔ **Fosinopril** (Monopril), available as 10, 20, and 40 mg tablets is usually started at a dose of 10 mg once a day rising to 80 mg at most. It may be necessary to divide the dose into two times a day if the blood pressure isn't low enough at the end of the single dose period. Fosinopril is broken down in the liver so that the usual dose can be given even when severe kidney disease is present.

✔ **Lisinopril** (Prinivil, Zestril) comes in many strengths: 2.5, 5, 10, 20, 30, and 40 mg. The starting dose is anywhere from 10 to 40 mg once a day. The kidneys eliminate Lisinopril from the body. The dose should be reduced if kidney function is poor.

Lisinopril also comes with hydrochlorothiazide as Zestoretic. It contains 10 mg of lisinopril and 12.5 mg of the diuretic, 20 mg/12.5 mg or 20 mg/ 25 mg. Prinzide contains the same two drugs in the same proportions.

✔ **Moexipril** (Univasc) is available as 7.5 and 15 mg tablets. The dose usually starts at 7.5 mg once a day taken at least an hour before a meal. The maximum dose is 30, which can be divided. Both liver disease and kidney disease prolong the activity of moexipril. The dose should be reduced in either case. Uniretic is moexipril and hydrochlorothiazide in the following proportions: 7.5 mg/12. mg and 15 mg/25 mg.

✔ **Perinopril** (Aceon), available in 2, 4, and 8 mg tablets, is usually started at a dose of 4 mg up to a maximum of 16 mg once a day. Doses should be reduced in the presence of decreased kidney function.

✔ **Quinapril** (Accupril) is supplied as 5, 10, 20, and 40 mg tablets. The starting dose is usually 10 mg a day, and the maximum is 80 mg once a day or divided. This drug doesn't reach its usual blood levels when taken with a high-fat meal. It's eliminated by the kidneys. The dose should be reduced if kidney failure is present.

Accuretic is a combination of quinapril with hydrochlorothiazide. The proportions are quinapril 10 mg and hydrochlorothiazide 12.5 mg, 20 mg/12.5 mg, and 20 mg/25 mg.

✔ **Ramipril** (Altace) is made in 1.25, 2.5, 5, and 10mg capsules. The dose is usually 2.5 mg to start, and the maximum dose is 20 mg once daily or divided up in two doses. Dosage should be adjusted downward in the presence of kidney disease.

✔ **Trandolapril** (Mavik) comes as 1, 2, and 4 mg tablets. The initial dose is usually 1 mg once daily adjusted up to 4 mg once daily. Dosage should be reduced in the presence of severe disease of the liver or kidneys.

Tarka is trandolapril plus verapamil. The proportions are 2 mg and 180 mg, 1 mg/240 mg, 2 mg/240 mg, and 4 mg/240 mg.

Why, you may ask, are all these different ACE inhibitors necessary? I don't know. ACE inhibitors aren't the drug of choice for high blood pressure but may be used when the diuretics or beta blockers can't be used for some reason. They're particularly useful in the presence of heart failure or diabetic kidney disease. They stand out by being free of most side effects.

How do you choose a particular one? That's a little easier to answer. One of the drugs that's taken once a day is probably better, although most of them need to be taken twice a day when the dose is raised. Your insurance company will probably dictate which one you use because they get a good price for that one (or two). That's as good a way as any to decide which drug to take, or if you have to pay for it directly, choose the cheapest drug.

Angiotensin II Receptor Blockers

These drugs, rather than blocking the enzyme as the ACE inhibitors do, block angiotensin II by not allowing it to attach to its receptor where it does its work of contracting arteries and releasing aldosterone. Because angiotensin II can be made by other enzymes besides angiotensin-converting enzyme, inhibition of angiotensin II by ACE inhibitors isn't complete. These receptor blockers can eliminate the activity of angiotensin II more completely. Drugs in this group all end with "artan".

Like the ACE inhibitors, these drugs are similar to one another. They've the advantage over ACE inhibitors in that they don't cause the dry cough. Recent studies of irbesartan and losartan show that they effectively reverse kidney disease in diabetes. This occurred even when the drug didn't lower the blood pressure much. They're relatively free of side effects although they can cause elevation in potassium because they're similar to the ACE inhibitors in their action. Occasional patients (less than 1 percent of those who take these drugs) develop headache or dizziness and have to discontinue the drugs. A rare patient develops facial swelling. Drug interactions don't seem to be a problem with this class.

These drugs don't change blood-fat levels, increase the uric acid, or increase the sugar in the blood. They are metabolized in the body into inactive substances, so elimination doesn't depend on the liver or the kidneys.

Like the ACE inhibitors, Angiotensin II receptor blockers shouldn't be prescribed for pregnant or breast-feeding women. Nor should it be prescribed for young women who plan to become pregnant soon.

The various drugs and their properties are as follows:

- **Candesartan cilexitil** (Atacand) comes as 4, 8, 16, and 32 mg tablets. The usual starting dose is 16 mg up to a maximum of 32 mg once a day. The dose does not need to be adjusted for mild liver or kidney disease.

- **Eprosartan** (Teveten) is available as 400 and 600 mg tablets. Starting at 400 mg once daily, the maximum dose is 800 mg once daily. The dose doesn't have to be adjusted for kidney disease or liver disease.

- **Irbesartan** (Avapro) is manufactured as 75, 150, and 300 mg tablets. Starting at 150 mg once a day, the dose goes up to 300 mg once a day.

  Avalide is irbesartan and hydrochlorothiazide. The proportions are 150 or 300 mg of irbesartan with 12.5 mg of hydrochlorothiazide.

- **Losartan** (Cozaar) was the first member of this class to be discovered. It comes as 25, 50, and 100 mg tablets. Treatment usually begins with 50 mg and goes up to 100 mg as a single dose or divided in half and taken twice a day.

  Hyzaar is losartan with hydrochlorothiazide. The dose is usually 50 mg losartan and 12.5 mg of the diuretic or 100 mg losartan and 25 mg of the diuretic.

- **Telmisartan** (Miscardis) is made in 40 and 80 mg tablets. The beginning dose is usually 40 mg once a day up to 80 mg once a day.

- **Valsartan** (Diovan) is produced in 80 and 160 mg capsules. Starting with 80 mg, the dose can go up to 320 mg once a day.

  Diovan HCT is valsartan plus hydrochlorothiazide. The proportions are 80 or 160 mg of valsartan plus 12.5 mg of hydrochlorothiazide.

Quick, make your selection before you have 12 other copies of the same drug to confuse you. In choosing one of these drugs, remember that they're not the first choice for high blood pressure therapy, except under the circumstances described earlier in this section. If you have the right to do it, ask for the one that's the least expensive and that can be taken once a day. The angiotensin II receptor blockers are about twice as expensive as the ACE inhibitors. Are they twice as good? It doesn't appear so. But for the person who cannot tolerate the cough caused by the ACE inhibitors, this may be a good solution.

Choosing a Drug

Now that you know all about the drugs that you can take to control your blood pressure, you're ready to put that information to use. Sure, your doctor makes the decisions about which medication to use, but you have the right to have some input, because that drug goes into *your* body, not your doctor's. Unfortunately, as brilliant as doctors are, doctors sometimes base their decisions on faulty information. Of course, it's never anything so obvious as which drug company representative is most alluring, but it could be something like which drug doctors are told about most often. In any case, our decisions should be based on evidence that a given drug is the best one for the situation.

Treating uncomplicated high blood pressure

Some basic principles for starting treatment follow:

1. Ideally, use a drug that can be given once a day, that's cheap, and has few side effects.

2. Start with a very low dose, maybe half the recommended dose; this is especially important for the elderly.

3. Increase the dose slowly until the desired effect is reached.

4. If the pressure isn't controlled at a reasonable dose, add a second drug with a different mechanism of action, or switch to another drug with a different mechanism of action. Again, start at a low dose and build up gradually.

5. If the drug isn't tolerated because of side effects, discontinue it, and try a drug with a different mechanism of action.

6. Always make sure that the patient has sufficient medication to last until the next appointment and that he has a return appointment before leaving the office.

7. Patient compliance, lack of which is the largest barrier to good treatment, is improved considerably if the patient understands exactly what the treatment is, what side effects to expect, and why it's necessary in the first place; hence, this book.

Medicating without fail

Here are some suggestions to make sure that you take your pills when you're supposed to:

✔ Get into the routine of taking the pills the same time each day.

✔ Associate pill-taking with another daily chore, such as brushing your teeth.

✔ Pills that need to be taken with food should be taken at the same meal daily.

✔ Post reminders all over the house where you can see them.

✔ Get a pill box and fill it daily, making sure it's empty at the end of the day.

This assumes that you don't have heart failure, eye disease, kidney disease, heart attacks, or other complications. Basically, you've gone to your doctor who has told you that your blood pressure is too high on several occasions and now wants to treat it after you've lost weight, started an exercise program, reduced your dietary salt, and tried one or several of the alternative treatments described in Chapter 12 without success.

Start with a diuretic, preferably hydrochlorothiazide, at a low dose of 12.5 or 25 mg daily. Give this at least two months to lower your blood pressure while getting your potassium checked occasionally. If the potassium falls abnormally low, add a potassium-sparing agent, probably amiloride.

Because higher doses don't seem to lower the blood pressure any better than low doses of hydrochlorothiazide, the next step, if necessary, is the addition of a beta-blocking drug. The one that has proven itself in clinical trials is propranolol. It's given in a starting dose of 20 mg twice daily. Some physicians recommend starting with a drug combination, such as Propranolol Hydrochloride and Hydrochlorothiazide Tablets and not bothering to use one drug. If the blood pressure is only mildly elevated, this isn't necessary.

Treating complicated high blood pressure

A number of different complications cause your choice to move away from the diuretics to some drug that can manage both the high blood pressure and the complication. The most important of these are discussed as follows:

- ✔ Heart failure is best treated by an ACE inhibitor and a diuretic. The diuretic in this case may not be one of the thiazide diuretics but the more powerful loop diuretics because too much fluid in the body is one of the major problems.

- ✔ Chest pain due to disease in the coronary arteries along with high blood pressure does better with beta blockers or calcium channel blockers.

- ✔ A heart attack with high blood pressure responds better to a beta blocker and an ACE inhibitor as the first choice. Although diltiazem and verapamil, calcium channel blockers, have shown the ability to reduce sickness and death in this situation.

- ✔ Diabetes mellitus with kidney disease and high blood pressure is best managed by an ACE inhibitor or one of the angiotensin II receptor blockers.

- ✔ Heart rhythm abnormalities with high blood pressure do better on beta blockers or calcium channel blockers, such as verapamil or diltiazem, but not nifedipine.

- Fat abnormalities in the blood along with high blood pressure are better treated with beta blockers that don't cause further fat abnormalities.

- Hand tremors along with high blood pressure may respond better to certain beta blockers, such as propranolol.

- If hyperthyroidism is present in addition to high blood pressure, a beta blocker is definitely the drug of choice.

- People with migraine headaches and high blood pressure do better with certain beta blockers or calcium channel blockers, such as propranolol or diltiazem.

- A person about to undergo surgery who has high blood pressure does better if the blood pressure medication during the surgery is a beta blocker.

When the first choice fails

If a prescription can't keep the blood pressure consistently under 140/90 mm Hg, further action must be taken. If it's because the blood pressure doesn't respond or the side effects are intolerable, a drug from another class is given. If the diuretics and beta blockers can't be used, the next step is an ACE inhibitor.

If the blood pressure is only partially controlled, a second drug from another drug class is added. If a diuretic hasn't been added, it should be added at this point. Then if the blood pressure still doesn't get down under 140/90 mm Hg, a third drug is added.

You should see your doctor again within one month after a change in medication.

Just because it took several drugs to bring your blood pressure under control doesn't necessarily mean that you're going to take all these drugs for the rest of your life. If you can lose weight or use some other method to bring down your blood pressure without drugs, you may be able to reduce dosages or stop some of the drugs. Even without other improvements, after a year of control, trying to cut down on some of the drugs under the care of your doctor is worthwhile.

The goal blood pressure for a person with diabetes or kidney disease is even lower than 130/85 mm Hg.

Recognizing Drug Side Effects

None of the drugs listed in this chapter are perfect; they all cause side effects and some of them are so severe that the drug must be discontinued. Being aware of side effects is important. If you notice an uncomfortable change shortly after you start a new drug for high blood pressure, it's relatively easy to know that the drug is to blame. Sometimes the side effect doesn't become apparent until months after you start the drug. At other times, the addition of another drug, often one that's used to treat another disease, brings out the side effect of the first drug. Look at the following list to see many of these side effects next to the blood pressure drugs that more commonly cause them.

If something in this list describes how you're feeling, discuss it with your doctor and consider a reduction in dosage or a change in the medication to a different class of drugs.

As a good rule of thumb, drugs in the same class have the same side effects. To rid yourself of an annoying side effect, you have to switch to a new class.

Side Effect	*Drug That May Cause It*
Anemia	Methyldopa
Breast enlargement	Spironolactone
Confusion	All diuretics
Constipation	Calcium channel blockers
Decreased good cholesterol	Beta blockers
Decreased white blood cells	ACE inhibitors
Depression	Clonidine, guanabenz, guanfacine, and calcium channel blockers
Diarrhea	Potassium-sparing diuretics
Dizziness	All diuretics, labetalol, and doxazocin
Dry cough	ACE inhibitors
Dry eyes	Clonidine, guanabenz, and guanfacine
Dry mouth	All diuretics, methyldopa, clonidine, guanabenz, and guanfacine
Fatigue	Beta blockers and doxazocin
Fever	Methyldopa, labetalol
Fluid in breasts	Methyldopa
Headache	Vasodilators and calcium channel blockers
Heart failure and vasodilators	Alpha-1 adrenergic receptor antagonists
Increased asthma	Beta blockers
Increased blood sugar	All diuretics
Increased cholesterol	Thiazide diuretics

Side Effect	*Drug That May Cause It*
Increased hairiness	Spironolactone and minoxidil
Increased urination	All diuretics
Irritation of the esophagus	Calcium channel blockers
Liver damage	Methyldopa
Loss of hearing	Loop diuretics
Loss of taste	ACE inhibitors
Lupus syndrome	Hydralazine
Menstrual irregularities	Spironolactone
Muscle pains	All diuretics
Nausea and vomiting	All diuretics
Rapid heart beat	Vasodilators
Reduced erections	Thiazide diuretics, spironolactone, and methyldopa
Skin rashes	All diuretics
Sleepiness	Methyldopa, clonidine, guanabenz, and guanfacine
Swelling of the abdomen	Potassium-sparing diuretics
Swelling of the legs	Vasodilators
Thirst	All diuretics
Very low blood pressure	ACE inhibitors
Vivid dreams or nightmares	Clonidine, guanabenz, and guanfacine
Weakness	All diuretics

These are the most common side effects identified with the drugs for high blood pressure. Many more less common problems are not listed here. If you have an unusual new symptom after starting a drug for high blood pressure, by all means, discuss it with your doctor and consider a reduction in dose or a change in medication.

Identifying Brand Names

So many drugs, so many brand names. How can you know what you're on, much less what it does and what its side effects may be? Doctors more often refer to a drug by its brand name because remembering the brand name is easier than remembering the scientific name. The drug companies want doctors to think of their drug when they write a prescription, so they give the drug a name that can stick in the mind, such as lotensin. The trouble is that the brand name only tells you what effect the drug has and often doesn't offer a clue as to what kind of drug it is.

In this section, I provide all the brand names of the current drugs in alphabetical order. Look up the brand name, and then refer to the drug's scientific name in the right column to find out what you're taking. You may discover that you're on a drug that you would be better off without, or it may explain that irritating symptom you've been having.

 Always keep an up-to-date list of all of your drugs, preferably by scientific and brand name. You should have the milligrams of the pill and the amount and frequency with which you take it. It can save your doctor plenty of time when prescription renewals are needed and any new doctor you see will know more about your health by the drugs you're taking.

 Some of these drugs are no longer made under their brand name because the patent has run out, and competing against a generic form of the drug is no longer profitable for the drug company. However, the doctor may still be using the brand name because he has always called it by that name, so you'll need to know the brand name anyway.

Brand Name	*Scientific Name*
Accupril	Quinapril
Accuretic	Quinapril and hydrochlorothiazide
Aceon	Perinopril
Adalat	Nifedipine
Aldactone	Spironolactone
Aldactazide	Spironolactone and hydrochlorothiazide
Aldoclor	Methyldopa and chlorothiazide
Aldomet	Methyldopa
Aldoril	Methyldopa and hydrochlorothiazide
Altace	Ramipril
Apresoline	Hydralazine
Apresozide	Hydralazine and hydrochlorothiazide
Aquatensen	Methyclorthiazide
Atacand	Candesartan cilexitil
Avalide	Irbesartan and hydrochlorothiazide
Avapro	Irbesartan
Blocardren	Timolol

Brand Name	*Scientific Name*
Bumex	Bumetanide
Calan	Verapamil
Capoten	Captopril
Capozide	Captopril and hydrochlorothiazide
Cardizem CD	Diltiazem
Cardura	Doxazosin
Cartrol Filmtab Tablets	Carteolol
Catapres	Clonidine
Clorpres	Clonidine and chlorthalidone
Combipres	Clonidine and chlorthalidone
Coreg	Carvedilol
Corzide	Nadolol and bendroflumethiazide
Covera	Verapamil
Cozaar	Losartan
Demadex	Torsemide
Dilicor XR	Diltiazem
Diovan	Valsartan
Diovan HCT	Valsartan and hydrochlorothiazide
Diuril Oral Suspension	Chlorothiazide
Diuril Tablets	Chlorothiazide
Dyazide	Triamterene and hydrochlorothiazide
Dyrenium	Triamterene
Edecrin	Ethacrynic acid
Enduron Tablets	Methyclorthiazide
HydroDIURIL	Hydrochlorothiazide
Hygroton	Chlorthalidone
Hytrin	Terzosin
Hyzaar	Losartan and hydrochlorothiazide
Inderal	Propranolol
Inderide	Propranolol and hydrochlorothiazide
Isoptin	Verapamil
Lasix	Furosemide

Brand Name	Scientific Name
Levatol	Penbutolol
Lexxel	Felodipine and enalapril
Loniten	Minoxidil
Lopressor	Metoprolol
Lotensin	Benazepril
Lotrel	Amlodipine and benazepril
Lozol	Indapamide
Mavik	Trandolapril
Maxide	Triamterene and hydrochlorothiazide
Midamor	Amiloride
Minipress	Prazosin
Minizide	Prazosin and polyzide
Miscardis	Telmisartan
Moduretic	Amiloride and hydrochlorothiazide
Monopril	Fosinopril
Mykrox	Metolazone
Naturetin	Bendroflumethiazide
Normodyne	Labetalol
Norvasc	Amlodipine
Oretic	Hydrochlorothiazide
Plendil	Felodipine
Prinivil	Lisinopril
Prinzide	Lisinopril and hydrochlorothiazide
Procardia	Nifedipine
Renese	Polythiazide
Sectral	Acebutolol
Sular	Nisoldipine
Tarka	Trandolapril and verapamil
Teczem	Diltiazem and enalapril
Tenex	Guanfacine
Tenormine	Atenolol
Teveten	Eprosartan

Brand Name	*Scientific Name*
Thalitone	Chlorthalidone
Tiazac	Diltiazem
Timolide	Timolol and hydrochlorothiazide
Toprol XL	Metoprolol
Trandate	Labetalol
Uniretic	Moexipril and hydrochlorothiazide
Univasc	Moexipril
Vasotec	Enalapril
Verelan	Verapamil
Wytensin	Guanabenz
Zaroxolyn	Metolazone
Zebeta	Bisoprolol
Zestril	Lisinopril
Zestoretic	Lisinopril and hydrochlorothiazide
Ziac	Bisoprolol and hydrochlorothiazide

Part IV
Investigating Special Populations

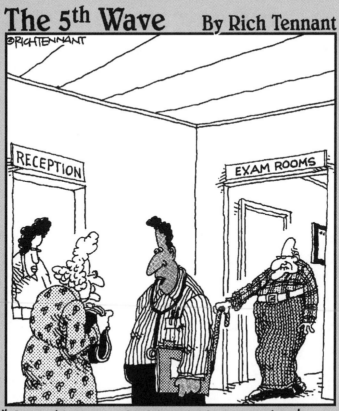

The 5th Wave   By Rich Tennant

RECEPTION   EXAM ROOMS

"Sometimes a tightness in the chest can be a sign of high blood pressure. In your husband's case, however, I just loosened his belt a little."

In this part . . .

Certain groups that may get high blood pressure require their own discussion. Certainly, children, the elderly, and the pregnant female have so many of their own issues that they deserve separate treatment. If you or a loved one is in one of these groups, you can find everything that you need to know about high blood pressure in this part.

Chapter 14

The Elderly

● ●

In This Chapter

▶ Taking care of those who can't care for themselves

▶ Finding out about an elderly person's high blood pressure

▶ Focusing on special nutritional needs and lifestyle changes

▶ Adding drugs to lower blood pressure

● ●

*W*ho are the elderly? It's a moving definition because more and more people are living longer and remaining healthier for a longer time. For the purposes of this chapter, let's consider the start of "elderly" to be age 75. The elderly are growing in numbers. The number of people living past 100 years of age is climbing. In the next thirty years, the concerns of the elderly will be a major challenge throughout the world. Don't be surprised if bathing suit ads start featuring 70-year-old grandmothers rather than 17-year-old girls!

The elderly are different from you and me. (Although I'm looking more and more like them.) Of course, some elderly are quite healthy; still, the elderly usually have more than one disease. They may have a certain amount of memory loss, which makes taking pills more challenging. The elderly are often on multiple medications with all the problems of drug interactions. Their nutrition may not be as good as it was at an earlier age. Their kidneys may have lost some of their function, and their vision may be poor. The elderly are at the greatest risk of a brain attack (see Chapter 7) or a heart attack, but controlling their blood pressure reduces this risk by at least 25 percent.

One important fact is that the incidence of high blood pressure among the elderly is enormous. Among individuals who are 75 years old on up, 75 percent of women and 65 percent of men have high blood pressure.

This chapter helps you understand the special problems of the elderly and how you can approach those problems, whether you're elderly or whether you have a loved one who is elderly with high blood pressure. As I write this, the Hypertension in the Very Elderly Trial is a key study going on in England to determine what effect blood pressure control has on the health of people 80 years of age and older. But plenty of information is available now to support the claim that blood pressure control does indeed affect the health of the elderly for the better. So if I were you, I wouldn't wait for the results of that study to bring your blood pressure or your loved one's blood pressure under control.

Evaluating Mental Disability

If a question exists as to an elderly person's ability to take medications, feed himself properly, and get physical exercise, then evaluating his mental ability is important. This can be done with a brief mental status examination performed by a doctor. This exam evaluates the following mental abilities:

- Orientation in time (day and year) and space (city and state)
- Ability to repeat items, read, write, draw, calculate, name items, and remember items previously named
- Comprehension

Standard versions of this test give an individual score; a perfect test receives a score of thirty. One version is the Mini-Mental State Examination. A person who scores less than 26 probably has some mental disability that can be further tested.

This is a good baseline test for any elderly person, not just one with high blood pressure. It can be repeated at intervals to observe deterioration. The test can also be used to determine if a loss of mental acuity is due to medication. And it takes just a few minutes to perform.

Your doctor should perform a brief mental status examination on your loved one at every office visit to look for indications that she can't care for herself.

If some degree of mental acuity is lost, medical care, especially the administration of drugs, shouldn't be left to the elderly individual. You or a healthcare professional — at home, in an assisted living facility, or nursing home — must take charge of medical care.

Assessing Blood Pressure

In the highly industrialized countries of the world, the systolic blood pressure rises throughout life. In contrast, the diastolic blood pressure begins to level off around age 55 or 60 and often falls after this leveling off occurs.

Dealing with essential high blood pressure

Almost all high blood pressure in the elderly is essential high blood pressure (high blood pressure for which the cause is unknown). Most of the high blood pressure in the elderly is also *isolated systolic high blood pressure,* which means that the systolic blood pressure is over 140 mm Hg, but the diastolic blood pressure is less than 90 mm Hg. In the elderly, systolic blood pressure can predict a brain attack or a heart attack. In fact, diastolic blood pressure elevation doesn't suggest the same risk as such an elevation would be in a younger person. Most often, *isolated diastolic high blood pressure,* where the systolic blood pressure is less than 140 mm Hg but the diastolic blood pressure is greater than 90 mm Hg, poses no more risk among the elderly than normal blood pressure. However, an individual with isolated diastolic blood pressure greater than 105 mm Hg probably needs some treatment, especially if complications of high blood pressure are present.

If you or a loved one is over 75 years of age with a systolic blood pressure reading that's greater than 140 on several occasions, you need some treatment, lifestyle change, or medication, to bring it down. Get together with your physician to set up a treatment plan.

Most of the time, an elderly person's high blood pressure is discovered during a routine examination or as part of a screening program put on by a local hospital or drugstore. About 10 percent of the time, the first indication of long-standing high blood pressure is found when a serious complication, such as a brain attack or a heart attack, occurs.

Pseudo high blood pressure is a condition resulting from the calcification of the arteries among the elderly. With aging, calcium is deposited along the artery, and this calcium may make it hard to compress the artery when the cuff around the arm is inflated during a blood pressure reading. The blood pressure meter registers high even though the blood pressure inside the artery is normal. The blood pressure may read as much as 20 to 30 mm Hg higher than its true value. A few clues can help to indicate that this condition is present:

- No sign of a high blood pressure complication presents itself even though the blood pressure is high.
- Blood pressure changes little despite giving adequate treatment.
- Low blood pressure symptoms are apparent while the measured blood pressure is normal or even still high.

A doctor can use techniques to get a direct measurement of blood pressure within the artery to evaluate the possibility of whether pseudo high blood pressure is present.

The benefits of controlling the blood pressure in the elderly are clear. A study in the *British Medical Journal* (January 1993) has shown that controlling the blood pressure in about 60 elderly people for five years can prevent one death due to a complication of high blood pressure. However, over two hundred younger people must have their blood pressure controlled for five years to prevent that one death.

Considering secondary high blood pressure

Secondary high blood pressure means that the high blood pressure is a direct result of a specific disease or disorder. If the disease disappears, then the high blood pressure is lowered. Treatment of the disorder often eliminates the high blood pressure. (Chapter 4 covers the various causes of secondary high blood pressure.) But an elderly person's high blood pressure is rarely due to another disease. Probably less than 1 percent of high blood pressure among the elderly is due to another disease or disorder. However, because curing that disease often cures the high blood pressure, it's worthwhile to consider the possibility under the following circumstances:

- Newly developed high blood pressure beyond 60 years of age
- Failure of three or more blood pressure drugs to control the blood pressure
- Symptoms or lab findings that suggest secondary high blood pressure (see Chapter 4)
- A low potassium level before drugs are used or with a small dose of a thiazide diuretic
- Continuing evidence of kidney function loss despite adequate blood pressure control

The steps to evaluate and treat the patient are in Chapter 4. Even though secondary high blood pressure may be found, curing the cause in the elderly, unless it developed recently, doesn't usually cure the high blood pressure. The blood pressure stays up even after eliminating a disease or disorder that causes high blood pressure because

- The high blood pressure has often been present for a long time.
- The elderly tend to have essential high blood pressure to begin with.

The kidney and other factors

More than likely, the diminishing function of one or both kidneys is responsible for blood pressure that's high. Blood flow to the kidney decreases by about 10 percent each decade after age 30 in a normal, healthy person. Circulation to the kidney is even less when high blood pressure, diabetes, or heart failure is present. Blood tests of kidney function may not reflect this decline because a test measures the excretion of creatinine, a chemical that comes from muscle. With aging, muscle mass decreases along with the blood flow into the kidney, so less creatinine needs to be excreted, and its level in the blood doesn't rise.

The main consequence of decreased blood flow to the kidney is the decreased ability of the kidney to get rid of salt and water in the body. This salt and water buildup causes the blood pressure to rise. Then the high blood pressure further decreases the kidney function. It's a vicious cycle.

Hormones coming from the adrenal gland (see Chapter 4), epinephrine and norepinephrine, are additional contributors to high blood pressure. Epinephrine raises blood pressure, heart rate, and blood glucose. Norepinephrine does the same thing. These hormones tend to be elevated in an elderly person's blood and don't fall as blood pressure rises.

The elderly also experience a defect in the production of nitric oxide in the walls of blood vessels. Nitric oxide is the most important chemical relaxant for the muscular walls of the arteries. Its absence leads to higher blood pressure.

Considering other things that elevate blood pressure in the elderly

Many elderly suffer from arthritis and receive *nonsteroidal anti-inflammatory drugs* (NSAIDs). These pain-reducing medications include ibuprofen (brand names Motrin, Advil), naproxen (Naprosyn), sulindac (Clinoril), diclofenac (Voltaren), piroxicam (Feldene), diflunisal (Dolobid), nabumetone (Relafen), etodolac (Lodine), oxaprozin (Daypro), indomethacin (Indocin), rofecoxib (Vioxx), celecoxib (Celebrex) and even aspirin in high doses of two aspirin taken three or more times a day. New NSAIDs come along on an almost daily basis. These drugs, especially when mixed with drugs for high blood pressure, block the action of the high blood pressure drug and raise the blood pressure.

An elderly person with high blood pressure taking an NSAID should discontinue the NSAID if possible, but only after consulting with her physician.

Of the NSAIDs, sulindac has been shown *not* to cause an increase in high blood pressure or to oppose the effect of blood pressure medications. This may be the drug of choice if an elderly individual — particularly an individual who has high blood pressure — needs an NSAID.

The *white coat effect* (see Chapter 2) is much greater in the elderly than the younger population. The white coat effect means that your systolic blood pressure may be 10 mm Hg higher when a physician takes the reading as compared to taking your blood pressure at home. An elderly patient may even have high blood pressure in the doctor's office and low blood pressure at home. For this reason, home blood pressure monitoring is a good idea for the elderly to determine if treatment is excessive or sufficient.

Improving Nutrition to Lower Blood Pressure

The goal of nutrition among the elderly is to provide the right amount of kilocalories from the appropriate energy sources with enough vitamins and minerals.

It may be helpful to take an elderly person to a supermarket and emphasize how food labels tell how much salt is found in various food products. Point out the best choices, which are usually the freshest foods.

Assessing diet

A dietary assessment determines whether an elderly person is getting enough of the right foods. One simple technique is to ask the person to write down everything that he eats for three days running. The memory of the older person limits this approach. A complementary approach is to ask the person to record how many times he eats a particular kind of food in a day, a week, or a month. A doctor can also measure blood levels of minerals and vitamins to determine if these nutrients are present in adequate amounts.

When a dietary assessment is done, an elderly individual's inadequate diet may turn up the following.

- ✔ Low vitamin and mineral intake
- ✔ Low fresh vegetable and fresh fruit intake
- ✔ Little variety in the diet
- ✔ Individual is underweight
- ✔ Frequent complaints of illness

The elderly with insufficient diets are often poor and uneducated, but inadequate diets are also found among the well heeled.

Because of the high cost of drugs and the lack of Medicaid or insurance coverage for prescriptions, many elderly claim that they must choose between good nutrition and their drugs. Although this economic problem is beyond the scope of this book, it's an important consideration. To be effective, high blood pressure treatment for the elderly must address both nutrition and drugs.

Following the DASH diet

The DASH diet, described in Chapter 9, is particularly valuable for the elderly, who don't get enough calcium in their diet. Elderly people who follow the DASH diet may reduce their blood pressure enough to eliminate a blood pressure medication. Because the side effects of drugs and drug interactions are a special problem, eliminating a drug is a goal worth having.

Another benefit of DASH is that it's low in saturated fat and cholesterol. Lowering fat and cholesterol contributes to the reduction of brain attacks and heart attacks in the elderly.

Energy needs decline with age, so kilocalorie intake must be reduced in the older population.

Reducing salt intake

Eating fresh foods and using herbs and spices in place of salt are essential for the elderly. The elderly are more sensitive to the blood-pressure-raising effect of salt than younger people. The more that salt intake is reduced, the greater the reduction in blood pressure.

When the DASH diet accompanies a reduction in salt intake, the result is even greater. Many elderly who follow DASH and reduce salt come off of all blood pressure medications. But reducing salt can be especially difficult for several reasons:

- ✔ The taste sensation is reduced, and the elderly may compensate by adding more salt to food.
- ✔ The elderly may live alone and not be able to consume fresh food before it spoils.
- ✔ They may lack the energy or ability to put their own food together.
- ✔ The elderly tend to consume more prepared foods, the very source of most of the salt in their diets.

Focusing on Lifestyle Changes to Lower Blood Pressure

Just as reducing salt intake tends to lower an elderly person's blood pressure more than it would in a younger individual, lifestyle changes also tend to lower an elderly person's blood pressure more than somebody younger. The most important changes include the following:

- Reducing alcohol intake is essential.

- Reducing weight can lower blood pressure enormously and reduce the risk of a heart attack.

- Quitting smoking is beneficial at any age.

- Increasing daily exercise has been shown to benefit the older person in many ways as well as lowering blood pressure. It reduces the chance of a fall, helps with weight loss, and adds strength to perform the tasks of daily living.

- A yoga program, meditation, or biofeedback may reduce blood pressure.

- If caffeine intake is more than two cups of regular coffee daily, this should be reduced.

Adding lifestyle changes to the proper diet goes a long way toward eliminating the need for drugs. In the Trial of Nonpharmacologic Interventions in the Elderly, a study in the *Journal of the American Medical Association* (March 1998), 975 men and women with high blood pressure between the ages of 60 and 80 were divided into four groups:

- **Salt reduction:** Cutting down to 1,800 mg of salt daily

- **Weight loss:** Losing at least ten pounds

- **Salt reduction and weight loss:** A combination of the salt reduction and weight loss group

- **Control:** A usual care group

After three months, 30 percent stopped all blood pressure medications. The group that lowered salt and reduced weight did best, but the salt reduction alone and weight loss alone groups still did much better than the control group. A key result is that the changes were sustained up to three years after the end of the study in these patients, even after decades of physical inactivity and unhealthy eating habits.

The National Long-term Care Survey, another study that can be found on the Internet at http://cds.duke.edu, paints an optimistic picture of disability, including high blood pressure, among the elderly in the future. Between 35,000 and 40,000 people have been studied at intervals of 2 to 5 years since 1982. The unexpected finding is that chronic disability among the elderly is falling at an increasing rate. Between 1982 and 1989, the prevalence of chronic disability fell at the rate of 1 percent per year. Between 1989 and 1994, it fell at 1.6 percent per year, and between 1994 and 1999, it fell at 2.6 percent per year. If this keeps up, by 2040, the prevalence of disability will be 50 percent of what it was in 2000. This means that despite a huge gain in the elderly population, the total number of disabled will be the same in 2040 as the year 2000. The main reason for this falling rate of chronic disability is the adoption of lifestyle changes among the elderly population. A second reason is the use of medical intervention.

This reminds me of an unlikely couple: an 80-year-old man who fell in love with a 20-year-old woman. She insisted that they get their health checked before considering marriage, and a doctor, after examining them both, told them they were in excellent health. "However," said the doctor, "I'm concerned about the age difference." The future husband replied, "Well, what can you do? If she dies, she dies."

Taking Drugs to Lower Blood Pressure

Some patients are unwilling or unable to make lifestyle changes. Even if they do change their habits, some patients still need to take drugs to get their blood pressure down to a level that doesn't cause illness or death. A number of basic recommendations are especially pertinent:

- An elderly person should take medication if the systolic blood pressure is 160 mm Hg or greater. The zone between 140 and 160 mm Hg is a gray area. Elderly people without complications of high blood pressure whose blood pressure is less than 160 mm Hg, don't benefit from treatment. However, if damage to the heart or blood vessels or a history of a brain attack is evident, then blood pressures over 140 but less than 160 mm Hg should be treated with drugs.

- Drug treatment should continue regardless of age as long as the patient is expected to live and side effects are mild.

- Other conditions, such as heart disease or diabetes, determine the - medication used.

- A once-daily medication is preferable to divided doses to achieve compliance with the drug regimen.

- Start with half the usual beginning dose for an elderly person. Make changes slowly to allow the person to become acclimated to the drug.

✔ Make sure the elderly individual can open the medication bottle and understands how to take the medication. Some safety bottles are impossible to open for people who have arthritis and/or vision problems.

✔ Drug interactions are a major potential problem because the elderly may be taking a number of prescription drugs.

Primary drug therapy: Thiazide diuretic

If an elderly person has uncomplicated high blood pressure, the first medication choice is a thiazide diuretic, which is the same drug that would be prescribed for a younger person without complications. But the elderly person would take half the usual dose. A dose of 12.5 mg of hydrochlorothiazide is effective in most elderly people. Going up to 50 mg is rarely necessary. Unfortunately, a pill that contains the 12.5 mg dosage isn't currently manufactured, so the elderly have to break the 25 mg pill in half.

Although the elderly often have high cholesterol, a harmful blood fat, this doesn't necessarily prohibit the use of a thiazide diuretic (which raises cholesterol at a high dose) at a low dose. The dose will probably have little effect on the cholesterol.

If the potassium or the sodium level is already low or the calcium is high, the thiazide diuretic can be combined with a potassium-sparing drug. Taking a potassium supplement isn't recommended for the elderly because the elderly have trouble both taking potassium by mouth and eliminating excessive potassium by the kidney.

Second choice: Beta blocker

If the patient can't take a thiazide diuretic or the drug isn't appropriate for some reason, a beta blocker is the second choice. Beta blockers are not as effective as thiazide diuretics, and beta blockers are associated with more side effects.

Beta blockers are less useful in elderly people who have congestive heart failure, asthma, chronic lung disease, or severe obstructive disease of the blood vessels. If the thiazide diuretic was used but didn't completely control the blood pressure, addition of a beta blocker often accomplishes a satisfactory blood pressure.

Third choice

Calcium channel blockers, ACE inhibitors, and angiotensin II receptor blockers (see Chapter 13) aren't as effective as a thiazide diuretic or a beta blocker but can be used when thiazide diuretics and beta blockers aren't appropriate for some reason, such as an allergy to the drugs. The trouble with the calcium channel blockers, ACE inhibitors, and angiotensin II receptor blockers is that although they definitely lower the blood pressure, they haven't been shown to reduce illness and death due to high blood pressure.

Medications prescribed for the treatment of high blood pressure can pose several dangers, such as the following:

- The danger of low blood pressure when an ACE inhibitor is added to a diuretic is great, especially in the elderly. The diuretic should be stopped for a few days before the ACE inhibitor is added.

- The initial dose of an ACE inhibitor must be reduced for an elderly person. If the usual starting dose is 10 mg, in the elderly person it should be reduced to 5 mg.

- The other classes of drugs that act on the brain, such as methyldopa, clonidine, guanfacine, and guanabenz as well as the alpha adrenergic receptor blockers, are powerful agents that cause drowsiness and depression as well as falls in blood pressure on standing. (See the "Special situations" section coming up.) They have limited use among the elderly population.

Special situations

Because chest pain associated with heart disease is so common in the elderly, using a beta blocker as the first choice of treatment is appropriate in the elderly person who has both chest pain due to coronary atherosclerosis (see Chapter 5) and high blood pressure.

ACE inhibitors have been shown to prolong the lives of those with congestive heart failure, so these would be the drugs of choice when heart failure accompanies high blood pressure.

ACE inhibitors and angiotensin II receptor blockers are especially good for the elderly person with high blood pressure who has kidney disease, which is often associated with diabetes.

Avoiding Dangerous Falls in Blood Pressure

In an elderly population, 10 percent may experience a sudden fall in blood pressure of 20 mm Hg or more after standing for one minute as compared to sitting down. This dramatic drop in blood pressure on standing is called *postural hypotension*. When the elderly have systolic high blood pressure, diabetes, or adrenal gland failure, the frequency of large falls in blood pressure on standing is even greater. The symptoms may include blurred vision, light-headedness, dizziness, and even a loss of consciousness.

Two tendencies account for an elderly individual's blood pressure to fall on standing:

- Blood tends to remain in the lower part of the body because of a loss of muscle tone and valves in blood vessels that ordinarily prevent blood backflow.
- The normal response of certain pressure sensors in the neck that detect when blood pressure falls is sometimes lost in the elderly.

  If functioning properly, these sensors send out signals to pump more blood into the brain. The heart pumps harder and blood vessels constrict to push blood back to the heart. However, if the sensors aren't functioning, the decreased blood in the brain may lead to a fainting spell or dizziness.

  Contributing to the reduction in blood flow to the brain may be the increase of blood in the intestinal blood vessels after eating.

A number of approaches treat falls in blood pressure on standing. Some of them include

- Tilting the bed to elevate the head
- Wearing elastic hose that reduce pooling of blood in the legs
- Leg exercises to push blood back to the heart
- It may be necessary to treat dehydration
- Adrenal medication to restore hormones missing in the event of an adrenal failure
- Reduction in the dose of blood pressure medication, particularly beta blockers and alpha blockers
- Conversely, sometimes controlling the blood pressure with drugs may reduce the tendency for a fall in blood pressure
- Certain drugs stimulate the blood vessels to contract

Chapter 15

High Blood Pressure Among Children

Children, like the elderly, are different from you and me. They're much smaller and still growing. Children are tuned into the opinions of their peers and usually don't like to be different. Having a chronic disease, such as high blood pressure, makes them stand out, and they don't want to. As a result, they may be unwilling to do what's necessary to manage their blood pressure, such as dieting and losing weight, reducing salt, and taking medications.

High blood pressure used to be a rare event in children. Now, as many as 10 percent of the population under the age of 18 may have high blood pressure. Although a child's high blood pressure may be due to any one of a number of causes, the major reason for high blood pressure's increasing incidence among children is that more and more kids are overweight or obese. A child is considered to be overweight if he is heavier than 85 percent of the children of the same age and height. The child is obese if he is heavier than 95 percent of the children of the same age and height. Your child's doctor should have charts that relate weight to age and height. Or you can go to the following site to find growth charts for boys and girl on the Internet: www.keepkidshealthy.com/growthcharts.

Even without an increase in high blood pressure, you can find out plenty if your child's blood pressure is checked periodically. Many believe that the roots of high blood pressure in adults can be found in children. If found and managed early enough, it may be possible to prevent adult high blood pressure.

In this chapter, you find all that you need to help prevent high blood pressure in your child and to manage it should your child have high blood pressure. Reward, praise, and encourage your child's positive efforts, however small, rather than punishing your child for *not* doing what she should. As the saying goes, you can get more bees with honey.

You might follow the example of the minister who needed his congregation to contribute more money to rebuild the church. He said to his parishioners, "Anyone willing to donate for the church fund, please stand up." At which point he had instructed his organist to play the Star Spangled Banner.

Measuring Blood Pressure Correctly

Just as in adults (see Chapter 2), proper measurement of a child's blood pressure is essential to make a correct diagnosis. This is especially challenging because the smallest child is unenthusiastic about having his arm wrapped in a cuff and squeezed while a stranger holds an instrument against his arm. This section shows you how to accomplish a proper blood pressure reading in any child.

Using Doppler ultrasound on tiny arms

Diagnosing high blood pressure is different for children. Size matters. Measuring blood pressure in the smallest infants and children with a stethoscope is difficult because the sounds are so hard to hear in their tiny arms. To overcome this problem, pediatricians use *Doppler ultrasound* instruments in place of a stethoscope to take blood pressure in the smallest arteries. Doppler was an Austrian who discovered that sound changed its pitch when it comes toward you as compared to when it's going away from you. If a sound wave is directed to an artery and a blood pressure cuff cuts off the blood flow, it bounces back with one sound wave appearance. When blood begins to flow through the artery as the cuff is deflated, the sound wave has a different appearance (this is the systolic blood pressure). As the cuff is opened further, the flow reaches its peak and the sound wave changes again (the diastolic blood pressure). The Doppler ultrasound instrument looks like a pencil held over the artery. It sends out sound waves that are altered by blood flow. The same "pencil" is connected to a machine that amplifies the altered sound wave of the artery, so you hear a distinct difference as blood flow starts.

Selecting the proper cuff size

The width of the blood pressure cuff must be appropriate for the size of the child's arm. If the cuff is too small, the blood pressure reading will be mistakenly high. If the cuff is too large, the blood pressure reading will be incorrectly low. Although the cuff itself must surround the upper arm completely, the length of the bladder — the part of the cuff that inflates with air — must cover at least 80 percent of the circumference of the upper arm. Its width should be 40 percent of the distance from the elbow to the shoulder. If a choice can be made between a cuff that appears a little small and the other a little large, use the larger cuff because it won't usually change the reading so much that high blood pressure is missed if present, while a small cuff usually produces a falsely elevated reading.

Using proper technique

Giving the child a chance to acclimate to the exam room before attempting a blood pressure reading is a good idea. A baby should be lying quietly and not sucking or crying. Whether the child is lying or sitting, the arm should be level with the heart. The right arm is conventionally used to measure blood pressure in children. If the child can sit, the child usually prefers sitting. If the blood pressure is elevated, measuring the blood pressure in both arms and the legs on the first visit is important.

In older children, usually beginning at age 3, the stethoscope can be used to measure the blood pressure in the conventional manner. The systolic blood pressure is the point at which sound is first heard as the cuff is deflated. The diastolic blood pressure is the point at which the sound disappears. (See the steps for taking a blood pressure reading in Chapter 2.)

If the blood pressure is high, the measurement should be repeated at least two other times on other occasions to confirm it.

Interpreting the Results of the Measurement

Children begin their lives with much lower blood pressure than later on. Understanding the progression of blood pressure in normal children is important. This can help you realize when blood pressure is too high. Blood pressure is dependent on height and weight, so these factors must be taken into account.

Normal blood pressure progression in children

At birth, the blood pressure of the newborn averages 70/45 mm Hg. Within a month, the systolic pressure rises to 85 mm Hg. After that, the blood pressure is normally up to about what you see in Table 15-1 according to the different age groups.

Table 15-1	Maximum Normal Blood Pressure at Different Ages
Age	*Blood Pressure*
Newborn	70/45 mm Hg
5	115/75 mm Hg
6–12	125/80 mm Hg
13–15	126/78 mm Hg
16–18	132/82 mm Hg
Over 18	139/89 mm Hg

Height can affect blood pressure. Normally, a taller child has higher blood pressure than a shorter child of the same age. The tallest child at age 10 may have a maximum blood pressure reading of 123/82 mm Hg while the shortest child at age 10 may have a maximum blood pressure reading of 114/77 mm Hg.

Finding abnormally high blood pressure

After the doctor is satisfied that the blood pressure is accurate, the blood pressure should be compared to the maximum blood pressure for a child of the same sex and height. Charts are available that the doctor can use to make this determination.

Children tend to be emotional in a doctor's office. The *white coat effect* (see Chapter 2) is often the reason for a child's elevated blood pressure. Home monitoring of blood pressure may help to rule out this problem.

The 90th percentile of blood pressure is the highest blood pressure that 90 percent of children of the same sex, height, and age may have. This can be found on children with blood pressures less than the 90th percentile are considered to have normal blood pressures. Children whose blood pressures are at the level of the 90th to the 95th percentile are said to have high-normal blood pressures. Children over the 95th percentile are considered to have high blood pressure. Thanks to the 1987 Task Force Report from the National Institute of Health and the National Heart, Lung, and Blood Institute, you can find the current tables that show the 90th and 95th percentile blood pressure levels for boys and girls ages 1 through 17 at various heights on the Web at www.nhlbi.nih.gov/health/prof/heart/hbp/hbp_ped.htm.

Because Table 15-1 shows the maximum normal blood pressures for different ages, they're actually the 95th percentile blood pressures. The 90th percentile blood pressures would generally be about 4 mm Hg lower, both systolic and diastolic. For example, if 126/78 mm Hg is the 95th percentile for children ages 13 to 15, 122/74 mm Hg is the 90th percentile. Children with blood pressures between those levels are considered high normal.

If your child has a blood pressure above the 90th percentile but below the 95th percentile, the blood pressure should be rechecked within three months. Generally, the repeat blood pressures will be normal.

Considering the Cause of Elevated Blood Pressure

Although the causes of high blood pressure in children vary, inheritance plays a role, and so does disease, and this section can help you better understand how high blood pressure develops in some children and not in others. Some factors, such as family history of high blood pressure, can be used to identify the children at high risk for high blood pressure as adults. The earlier that preventive measures can be taken, the greater the likelihood that the child will not develop high blood pressure as an adult. The future of quality high blood pressure care lies in prevention.

Hereditary influences

Genetics undoubtedly influences the development of high blood pressure. If a parent has high blood pressure, one third of her children are likely to develop high blood pressure as well. If both parents have high blood pressure, two out of three children are likely to develop high blood pressure.

Children who may have high blood pressure as adults because their parents have high blood pressure react differently to many challenges than those children who do not have parents with high blood pressure. Children born to parents with high blood pressure may

- Experience an excessive rise in blood pressure after exercise
- Respond to emotional stress with a much greater rise in blood pressure
- Often have increased plasma renin activity
- Have a greater rise in pulse rate than usual during exercise
- Respond to a mental challenge, such as a school test, with a rise in blood pressure

These abnormalities are especially striking in children from ethnic groups that have the highest prevalence of high blood pressure, especially African Americans.

Usually, if parents with high blood pressure adopt a child, the child won't develop high blood pressure unless at least one biological parent had it. If one identical twin has high blood pressure, the other will have it more than 50 percent of the time, but if a fraternal twin has high blood pressure, the other will have it less than 50 percent of the time.

Factoring in weight

Of the factors that affect high blood pressure early in life and in the child's future, an overweight or obese childhood is significant. At any age, a strong relationship exists between weight and blood pressure.

Newborns who have a low birth weight tend to have higher blood pressures by the time they're adolescents than those who have normal weight at birth. Even when the overweight condition doesn't continue into adulthood, the adult who was overweight as a child has a higher rate of heart illness as an adult. These children eat more salt than their peers who are without high blood pressure do.

If an overweight child loses weight, however, she often reverses her high blood pressure.

Resulting from disease

When a newborn or a child up through 6 years of age has high blood pressure, it's usually secondary high blood pressure — the result of a disease. The most common causes of secondary high blood pressure among newborns and children up through 6 years of age are kidney disease, blockage of one or both arteries to the kidney, or coarctation of the aorta. These causes are discussed in Chapter 4.

Beginning at age 7, essential high blood pressure (high blood pressure for which the cause is unknown) begins to appear, although it's still rare at this age. Kidney disease and blockage of the kidney arteries are still found as frequent causes of secondary high blood pressure in this group. Elevated blood pressure due to overweight and obese conditions also begins to become important at this age.

By age 11, essential high blood pressure is becoming more prevalent along with kidney disease. These children are beginning to look more like adults in the spectrum of causes for high blood pressure. Before this age, up to 90 percent of the children have secondary high blood pressure (high blood pressure that's symptomatic of a disease).

Pinpointing the Cause of the Elevated Blood Pressure

If you discover that your child has high blood pressure, your child must undergo a careful evaluation because the cause is most often secondary to a known disease, which may be reversible. The doctor's evaluation should include a careful history of the child and the family, a physical examination emphasizing possible causes of high blood pressure, and appropriate laboratory studies that may point to a cause.

Key points in the history

Because of high blood pressure's hereditary connection, finding out from the parents whether high blood pressure is present in parents, grandparents, and close relatives is important. A family history of obesity is predictive of high blood pressure in the child. If brothers and sisters of the child also have high blood pressure, then a genetic basis for the high blood pressure may be established.

The child may have a history of some illness that could damage the kidneys, such as repeated infections of the kidney or bladder. An important clue to the cause of high blood pressure in the older child is the abuse of legal drugs like amphetamines or the use of illegal drugs like cocaine. These drugs can be detected in blood tests.

Finding out about what your child eats is essential. See whether he eats many packaged foods that may be high in kilocalories and salt.

Clues discovered during the physical examination

Getting an accurate pulse is also important. The pulse rate may suggest an excess of certain hormones if it's rapid. An accurate height and weight allows the doctor to place the blood pressure in the correct percentile. Of course, it's sometimes difficult to get the correct weight of a small child. But you might take the clerk's suggestion in the story that follows:

At a pharmacy, a young woman asked to use the infant scale to weigh the baby she held in her arms. The clerk explained that the device was out for repairs, but he suggested that the mother could figure the infant's weight by weighing herself together with the baby on the adult scale, and then the mother could weigh herself alone. To find the baby's weight, the second weight could be subtracted from the first. "But that's impossible," countered the woman, "I'm not the mother; I'm the baby's aunt."

Some of the other important features of the physical examination in the child from age 1 to 18 include:

- ✔ The blood pressure is taken in both arms and legs when it's elevated. A large difference suggests coarctation of the aorta.

- ✔ The physical appearance of the child may suggest a diagnosis of Cushing's syndrome (see Chapter 4). A round flushed face and pigmented stretch marks may be present, for example.

- ✔ The doctor should listen carefully for humming sounds over the arteries to the kidneys and the aorta. If found, these sounds suggest obstruction to the flow of blood.

- ✔ A careful eye examination can show any changes associated with high blood pressure.

- ✔ Abnormal function of the thyroid gland may be a cause of high blood pressure and the size and texture of the gland should be carefully observed and felt.

- ✔ The heart is examined for damage due to high blood pressure, particularly enlargement.

- ✔ The abdomen is felt for the presence of masses that might suggest a tumor.

Getting help from the laboratory

If one of the secondary causes of high blood pressure is clearly suspected, the specific lab tests noted in Chapter 4 should be done. If not, several tests may point to a specific diagnosis:

- Examination of the urine can reveal the infection that leads to kidney damage. A urine exam can also show the presence of blood and excess protein, which may indicate that the kidneys are leaking abnormally.

- Because kidney damage is frequently the cause of secondary high blood pressure in younger children, an ultrasound study of the kidneys shows the size and shape of the kidneys as well as any appearance of disease.

- Blood levels of chemicals for kidney function are helpful.

- A blood potassium level can help to rule out a rare aldosterone-making tumor.

After this complete evaluation is performed, a doctor can find the cause in most children. If it's something reversible, such as obstruction of a kidney artery or coarctation of the aorta, then surgery is needed. Something irreversible, such as a damaged kidney, can at least be slowed down by treating the high blood pressure with lifestyle changes and, if necessary, medication.

Beginning Treatment with Lifestyle Changes

Making lifestyle changes can control high blood pressure. This may be all that's necessary to reverse high blood pressure in many children, especially older children. The various steps include the following:

- **Losing weight:** If the child is overweight, a great effort should be made to help the child lose weight. This is best done by carefully evaluating the current diet and altering it to eliminate obvious sources of empty kilocalories, such as sodas, reducing sources of saturated fat and cholesterol, and reducing portions of all foods to get the total kilocalorie intake low enough to produce a slow but steady weight loss. But don't deprive the child of the joys of eating completely. A hamburger or pizza can fit into such a diet if not eaten to excess.

- **Reducing salt:** Salt reduction is key to lowering blood pressure. The child can discover how to enjoy the taste of other foods that are not salty. This is essential to promote lifelong control of salt intake.

Managing salt at this stage may prevent high blood pressure as the child becomes an adult. In addition to reducing salt, diets that raise the potassium can lower the blood pressure even more. Foods that are especially high in potassium include beet greens, broccoli, cauliflower, carrots, lettuce, spinach, tomatoes, bananas, and oranges.

✔ **Choosing healthy foods:** Encourage the child to follow a diet made up of increased amounts of fruits and vegetables, that's low in fats, and has more servings of grains. The DASH diet (see Chapter 9), lowers the blood pressure in the normal weight child as well as the overweight child.

✔ **Exercising:** Exercise is another key to lifelong high blood pressure prevention. The child needs to understand that moving the body is as crucial to lifelong health as eating properly. You can find out more about exercise in the following section because some question exists about the relationship between strenuous exercise and high blood pressure in children.

✔ **Avoiding stress:** If stress is playing a role in the high blood pressure, this must be addressed as well. The child may need some brief therapy to deal with his fears and concerns about having a disease that none of his buddies have to deal with.

✔ **Quitting coffee:** A child who drinks coffee with caffeine should be encouraged to give it up. It's another habit that's easily taken into adulthood but can be eliminated if dealt with at a young age.

✔ **Quitting tobacco:** Tobacco in any form should be forbidden, whether it's smoked, snuffed, or chewed. A child who may only have smoked for a fairly brief period will have a much easier time stopping than the person who has had the habit for years. Parents must be clear on this point and need to set an example by quitting if the parent is a smoker. It's ridiculous for a parent to go on smoking while sermonizing their child on the dangers of tobacco use.

✔ **Controlling diabetes:** If the child has diabetes, controlling the blood glucose can help to control blood pressure.

Some of the points discussed in the preceding list can lower blood pressure but medication for the diabetes may be required as well.

Advising the Child About Strenuous Exercise

Many children want to engage in strenuous exercise and sports and don't want high blood pressure or any other abnormality to prevent them from doing so. In the absence of *severe high blood pressure* or damage to the eyes, kidneys, or heart, children can do just about any form of physical exercise that they desire. In general, combining boys and girls together and not considering height, severe high blood pressure means a blood pressure greater than 129/85 mm Hg for ages 6 through 9, greater than 133/89 mm Hg for ages 10 through 12, greater than 143/91 mm Hg for ages 13 through 15, and greater than 149/97 mm Hg for ages 16 through 18.

If severe high blood pressure is present, then children shouldn't be permitted to participate in competitive sports or sports that require a great deal of physical exertion over a short period of time, such as bodybuilding, rowing, and boxing, until the blood pressure is brought under control, and evidence of damage to their eyes, kidneys, or heart, is nonexistent. However, less strenuous activities, such as jogging, are permissible.

If high blood pressure and a disease of the heart or the blood vessels are present, the severity of the heart or blood vessel disease determines what they are allowed to do.

Any athlete, but especially the athlete with high blood pressure, should avoid drugs that supposedly build up the muscles or energy, such as growth hormone, cocaine, tobacco, alcohol, and excessive salt. It may be illegal for athletes in particular sports to use some of the mainstays in the treatment of high blood pressure, especially diuretics and beta blockers. They need to use other medications that aren't banned by their sport. The bottom line is that high blood pressure doesn't shut the door to athletic performance but it must be done wisely, especially if the blood pressure is severe and/or damage to the eyes, kidneys, or heart occurs.

Using Drugs

The treatment of children with high blood pressure when drugs are necessary is similar to the treatment of adults. Mild high blood pressure is treated with a low dose diuretic (see Chapter 13), equivalent to 12.5 mg of hydrochlorothiazide. If it's necessary to add a second drug, a beta blocker (also discussed in Chapter 13) is most often used.

If the combination of a diuretic and a beta blocker don't control blood pressure in these children, an ACE inhibitor, an angiotensin II receptor blocker or a calcium channel blocker (all discussed in Chapter 13) can be used. If possible, using a single agent is always best because children are reluctant to take one pill a day, much less one pill two or three times a day.

Prior to starting drug treatment and while the child is taking the drug, frequent monitoring is important, both to check the effect and to be sure the child is actually taking the medication. This is where a parent can be helpful at home, checking the blood pressure every few days. Most children, after they're forced to take a pill every day, will gladly start to make changes in lifestyle, such as a reduction in food intake, a reduction in salt or an increase in exercise, that may result in an elimination of the pill.

To see if taking medication can be discontinued permanently, stopping blood pressure medication after a year or so of successful blood pressure control is worthwhile. Ask your child's doctor if the medication can be stopped for a brief period of time to evaluate whether the blood pressure elevation persists after a year of successful control.

Chapter 16

Women and High Blood Pressure

. . . .

In This Chapter

▶ Discovering prenatal changes that affect blood pressure

▶ Finding out about preeclampsia, eclampsia, and the HELLP syndrome

▶ Delivering a baby and reducing the risk to the mother-to-be

▶ Taking hormones during menopause

. . . .

*P*roviding medical care to a pregnant woman (so far, I haven't helped any pregnant men) is one of the more gratifying activities of a physician. You start out with a happy woman and end up with a thrilled woman and a healthy new life — that is, most of the time. On occasion, I have run into medical problems, such as high blood pressure, associated with a pregnancy.

High blood pressure may appear before a pregnancy or during the pregnancy and may be temporary or permanent. Most of the time, high blood pressure management during pregnancy is simple and straightforward. It's rare that the pregnant woman suddenly develops signs and symptoms around the middle of the pregnancy that put her and her growing fetus at risk for sickness and even death. Fortunately, this complication called preeclampsia (discussed later in this chapter in the "Preeclampsia" section) has become unusual, but it still happens, and you need to be aware of it if you're the pregnant woman, the future father, or a caring friend or relative.

In this chapter, you discover the different ways that high blood pressure develops during pregnancy, how to differentiate between the various causes, and what needs to be done about it. Hopefully, you'll come away from reading this chapter with a greater appreciation for the miracle of birth and a good understanding of high blood pressure management when it complicates this miracle.

Understanding How a Woman's Blood Pressure Responds to Pregnancy

Blood pressure isn't the same during a pregnancy as before the pregnancy. The pregnant woman's body goes through many changes to provide the best possible environment for the growing fetus. The mother-to-be must sustain the placenta and the umbilical cord (the connection between the mother and the fetus) as well as the fetus itself with nutrition and fluid. To do this, the expectant mother's blood vessels widen, and the volume of water and salt increases in her body. She gains about eight liters (two gallons) of water.

The effect of the opening of blood vessels on the blood pressure is that it normally falls during the first six months of the pregnancy. Even the woman who has pre-existing high blood pressure may be able to stop high blood pressure medications during pregnancy because the blood pressure may drop into the normal range.

If you have high blood pressure before you become pregnant, have your doctor check your blood pressure after you become pregnant to see if you can reduce or stop blood pressure medication. Also, if you suffer from kidney disease, the risk of kidney failure increases significantly during pregnancy. Potential mothers should discuss whether pregnancy is advisable with their doctor before becoming pregnant. For this reason, be sure to get a complete medical evaluation for any evidence of target-organ damage (damage to the organs that high blood pressure affects, especially the heart, kidneys, and eyes). For more on target-organ damage, see Chapter 8.

Normal hormonal changes during pregnancy

During pregnancy, the production of various hormones increases to foster fetal growth as well as to sustain and prepare the mother-to-be for delivery and breast-feeding. The production of renin, an enzyme made by the kidney whenever it detects a fall in blood pressure, is also increased (see Chapter 4) during pregnancy. This increase may be because of the increase in blood volume but also because the placenta makes renin as well. Estrogen, progesterone, and prolactin — all hormones — also increase their production during pregnancy. The estrogen may be responsible for some of the increased blood flow. Prolactin increases in preparation for breast-feeding. A new hormone called relaxin from the placenta also helps to open blood vessels.

Recognizing What Causes High Blood Pressure During Pregnancy

Several different factors cause high blood pressure during pregnancy. Differentiating between high blood pressure that began before the pregnancy from high blood pressure that starts during the pregnancy is important. The consequences are completely different.

Chronic high blood pressure

A woman with chronic high blood pressure has a blood pressure of more than 140/90 mm Hg on repeated occasions, and it's present before pregnancy or recognized before the 20th week of the pregnancy. Because so many women haven't had their blood pressure measured before a pregnancy and because blood pressure falls normally during the first six months of a pregnancy, chronic high blood pressure may go unnoticed until the final three months of the pregnancy.

As noted previously, it may be possible to stop blood pressure medication in a woman with chronic high blood pressure during early pregnancy. After it's stopped, it may be better for the pregnancy not to start taking the blood pressure medication again until the baby is born. Evidence that the outcome of the pregnancy is improved if the mother's blood pressure is treated for the short duration of a pregnancy doesn't exist. However, if the diastolic blood pressure is above 100 mm Hg or damage to the heart or the kidneys of the mother is known, the medication should be given.

The favorite medication for high blood pressure during pregnancy is methyldopa (see Chapter 13). Safe for both the mother and the growing fetus, methyldopa is very effective. If the woman is already on a diuretic (see Chapter 13), it can be continued, but it should not be started during the pregnancy because it tends to lower the blood volume, which needs to be greater during a pregnancy. If methyldopa is ineffective, another drug that has been successful is labetalol. The angiotensin-converting enzyme (ACE) inhibitors and the angiotensin II receptor blockers are both dangerous to the fetus and must be stopped as soon as a woman becomes pregnant, preferably earlier.

If you're pregnant and have high blood pressure, become familiar with the drugs in Chapter 13. Don't take any of the ACE inhibitors or the angiotensin II receptor blockers because both endanger the fetus.

A woman who begins a pregnancy with a diagnosis of chronic high blood pressure won't want to do strenuous exercise during the pregnancy. The risk to the fetal blood supply is too great.

Chronic high blood pressure poses increased risks to the mother and the fetus. These risks are even more dangerous in African American women and those with diastolic blood pressure over 110 mm Hg. The main ones are:

- A greater risk of developing preeclampsia (discussed in the following section).

- Increased danger of disease and death for the fetus, such as retarded growth of the fetus when the mother has chronic high blood pressure. This must be monitored with monthly ultrasound studies.

- Possible significant worsening of the mother's kidney function if kidney disease is present.

Preeclampsia

Preeclampsia is high blood pressure associated with symptoms such as headache, weight gain, blurred vision, swelling, and abdominal pain beginning after the 20th week of the pregnancy. Preeclampsia, if unchecked, can lead to seizures. Although its cause is unknown, preeclampsia is found in roughly 5 percent of all pregnancies in most advanced nations and to a higher degree in more disadvantaged countries. Dangerous for both the fetus and the mother, preeclampsia doesn't begin until the 20th week of the pregnancy, and delivering the baby and the placenta usually cures it. You're at higher risk of developing preeclampsia if you're a woman who is

- Having your first baby (especially, if you're older than 40 or younger than 19) or your first baby with a new partner.

- Carrying a twin pregnancy.

You're also at higher risk of developing preeclampsia if you're a woman who has

- High blood pressure already

- Diabetes with diabetic complications, such as eye disease, kidney disease, or nerve disease (See *Diabetes For Dummies* by yours truly [Wiley].)

- Any pre-existing kidney disease before becoming pregnant

- Had preeclampsia in a previous pregnancy

- A mother with preeclampsia

Attempting to prevent preeclampsia

Preeclampsia can't be prevented, and several treatments haven't worked that were used in the past. Anything the mother-to-be can do to remain in the best health possible can help should preeclampsia develop.

Anything that harms the fetus and the mother should be eliminated so as not to worsen the prospects for the pregnancy. In that respect, both tobacco and alcohol must be stopped at the beginning of a pregnancy if not before. (See Chapter 11 for more on quitting tobacco and alcohol use.)

An important factor in the development of preeclampsia is the production of chemicals that constrict arteries enough to raise blood pressure and inhibit chemicals that open arteries. It was thought that aspirin may be useful. Aspirin can inhibit the constricting chemicals, but aspirin hasn't caused a decrease in cases of preeclampsia when compared with women who didn't get aspirin.

Calcium was also suggested because its use seemed to reduce the occurrence of preeclampsia, but it has not proved to be helpful either. Calcium doesn't reduce the cases of preeclampsia or delay the beginning of the condition.

Diagnosing preeclampsia

Preeclampsia is usually diagnosed when the blood pressure rises to 140/90 mm Hg after the 20th week and excessive levels of protein are discovered in the urine. (But protein isn't always found in the urine as a result of preeclampsia.) Protein loss usually accompanies swelling of the expectant mother's body, but swelling is so common during pregnancy that it's not used to diagnose preeclampsia. Usually, the expectant mother with preeclampsia experiences some or all of the following symptoms:

- ✔ Abdominal pain
- ✔ Abnormal liver enzymes in the blood
- ✔ Blurred vision
- ✔ Excessive and rapid weight gain
- ✔ Headache
- ✔ Low platelet counts in the blood resulting in abnormal clotting and bleeding
- ✔ Nausea

If your doctor suspects that you have preeclampsia, ask her to treat you as though you do have it even if she isn't certain of the diagnosis. Preeclampsia is one condition that should be overdiagnosed because the results can be so devastating for the mother and the fetus. Also, as in any diagnosis of high blood pressure, more than one measurement of blood pressure should be taken. But because this is a serious and dangerous disease, the measurements should be no more than a few days or even hours apart.

Some pregnant women exhibit certain signs of preeclampsia but don't have high blood pressure. This condition is the *HELLP syndrome.* HELLP is an acronym that stands for hemolytic anemia, elevated liver enzymes, and low platelets. Women who experience headache, nausea, and pain in the abdomen during pregnancy may have the HELLP syndrome — a serious condition that disappears after delivery of the baby most of the time.

Worsening preeclampsia

As preeclampsia gets worse, some or all of its signs and symptoms become more severe and new symptoms develop. Headaches become more persistent and painful; restlessness increases; pain over the stomach worsens. Among the new findings are

- Development of anemia (low red blood cell count) because of the breaking up of red blood cells (hemolysis)

- Broken pieces of red blood cells called *schistocytes* on a blood smear indicate that red blood cells are being broken up

- Increasing kidney failure

- Increasing levels of uric acid in the blood. Normally, uric acid falls in early pregnancy while it's higher in cases of preeclampsia.

- Increased blood clotting demonstrated by blood tests of clotting

- Heart failure in the mother

- Any suggestion of a rupture of the placenta with bleeding

- Abnormal nonstress test of the fetus. The nonstress test consists of measuring the rate of the fetal heart when it moves. A heart rate that doesn't increase with fetal movement is abnormal.

- Evidence of reduced fetal growth

At this point, the situation is extremely serious and treatment must be administered rapidly. This isn't a situation that can be managed outside the hospital without the aid of an experienced physician.

Treating preeclampsia

One form of treatment that cures the preeclampsia is termination of the pregnancy. If the pregnancy is at 36 weeks or longer, delivery can take place immediately. However, the fetus may not be mature enough to survive if the pregnancy hasn't continued to at least the 28th week. Therefore, if no signs appear that the preeclampsia is worsening to the point that the mother's life is in danger, an attempt is made to prolong the pregnancy as much as possible. Each extra day means a great deal for the safe delivery of the baby.

Some of the steps that the doctor can take to avoid early delivery include:

✔ Lowering the blood pressure so that it's between 90 and 110 mm Hg diastolic. This is often done with medications given in the vein of the mother for an immediate effect.

✔ Giving magnesium sulfate into the vein of the mother to prevent convulsions, the complication that turns preeclampsia into eclampsia

✔ Constant monitoring of the mother with blood pressure measurements, weights, checking of fetal movements and measuring of urine protein.

✔ Complete bed rest for the mother if the preeclampsia is more severe.

✔ Continuation of a good diet with no reduction in salt to avoid further decreasing the blood volume of the mother

When these steps are taken, most mothers avoid moving from preeclampsia to eclampsia (discussed in the following "Dealing with eclampsia" section), and the complications of preeclampsia for the mother and the fetus can be prevented as well.

Theories on how preeclampsia develops

Although how preeclampsia occurs is unknown, one of the initiating events, if not the cause, is the failure of tissue from the placenta to achieve the normal amount of connection with blood vessels in the uterus called the spiral arteries. The result is that the fetus doesn't receive sufficient nutrition. This poor connection has a greater tendency to occur in a twin pregnancy that's complicated by hydatidiform moles (fluid-filled cysts that replace the placenta and fetus), diabetes, and a prior history of high blood pressure.

Detecting inadequate blood supply to the fetus, the placenta begins to produce more of a hormone that raises blood pressure by constricting arteries and less of a hormone that lowers blood pressure by opening arteries. One result is a rise in blood pressure. Other chemical factors are produced that are responsible for the other findings: increased sclotting and liver damage.

Preeclampsia is probably hereditary because it's found more often in the daughters of mothers who had it.

Another suspected contribution to the development of preeclampsia is the body's immune system. In a normal pregnancy, the mother's immune system doesn't reject the tissue of the fetus, which is really foreign to the mother and would be expected to be rejected under other circumstances. In preeclampsia, the mother's immune system is rejecting the fetal tissue to some extent. The incidence of preeclampsia is lower if the mother-to-be has had prolonged sexual contact with the father prior to the pregnancy. Thus, the expectant mother is exposed to his tissues, and her body has become accustomed to the foreign tissue that the fetus contains.

The best route for the baby's delivery is through the vagina. This eliminates the added stress of surgery. The mother is given an anesthesia by way of a needle in the lower back, the epidural or spinal space rather than general anesthesia, which can bring on increased blood pressure as a breathing tube is inserted and removed.

After the baby is delivered, the mother's abnormalities should disappear in a few days or weeks unless the injury to certain organs, such as the kidneys, has been severe in which case organ damage may be permanent. Testing over time can determine this.

The risk is low for the development of preeclampsia in future pregnancies, if organ damage isn't permanent. The mothers don't usually suffer from permanent high blood pressure.

Dealing with eclampsia

If the mother-to-be with preeclampsia has convulsions, the condition is *eclampsia.* Fortunately, it occurs rarely — only about once in every 2 thousand pregnancies — but it can threaten the life of the mother and the fetus.

Eclampsia results from severe narrowing of the blood vessels in the brain of the mother so that the supply of nutrients to the brain cells is diminished. Convulsions usually take place before the baby is delivered, but convulsions have occurred after delivery, too. High blood pressure doesn't necessarily have to be present when convulsions occur. One out of five patients has a blood pressure of less than 140/90 mm Hg just before convulsing.

The convulsions don't always take place conveniently in a hospital setting. If they occur at home, it's essential to know how to deal with them to the extent that you can. Turning the mother on her side can help to prevent taking the contents of the stomach into the lungs as well as improving blood flow to the placenta. A padded stick is inserted into the mouth to prevent biting the tongue. This is clearly an emergency requiring a 9-1-1 call and transportation to the hospital.

After the patient arrives in the hospital or if the convulsions occur in the hospital, magnesium sulfate is given into her vein to stop the convulsions. Then the blood pressure is controlled if necessary, again with medication into the vein. At the same time, the fetus is being monitored.

When everything appears to be more stable, delivery of the baby is carried out. It's preferred that delivery take place through the vagina but Cesarean section is performed if the most rapid delivery is desired.

After the baby is delivered, the magnesium sulfate is continued for several days until the signs of preeclampsia and eclampsia are clearly diminishing. A good indicator is the beginning of the excretion of the large amount of extra body fluid that the mother has accumulated.

Just like the situation for preeclampsia, the prospects for a mother who has had eclampsia are good for a future pregnancy or the development of permanent high blood pressure. Having eclampsia in a later pregnancy is unusual. Women who have had eclampsia have no more high blood pressure later on than women who've never had eclampsia.

Preeclampsia on top of chronic high blood pressure

When preeclampsia complicates chronic high blood pressure during a pregnancy, the risks for the mother and the fetus are greater than the risks for either condition alone. It may be difficult to tell whether the chronic high blood pressure is getting worse or preeclampsia has begun to occur. A number of studies point to the onset of preeclampsia on top of chronic high blood pressure. The most useful of these are

- Finding protein in the urine when protein hasn't been found in the urine previously
- A sudden increase in protein in the urine
- A sudden increase in high blood pressure that has previously been controlled
- Finding a platelet count in the blood of less than 1 hundred thousand per cubic millimeter
- Discovering abnormal liver function as the result of tests

The treatment of preeclampsia in association with chronic high blood pressure must be even more attentive than the treatment of preeclampsia alone. The decision to end such a pregnancy is made even earlier than when there is no complicating chronic high blood pressure.

Gestational high blood pressure

High blood pressure known as *gestational* (associated with a pregnancy) is *transient high blood pressure*. If no preeclampsia is associated with the pregnant woman's high blood pressure and the high blood pressure disappears 12 weeks after delivery or chronic high blood pressure is present (if the high blood pressure doesn't go away), then it's a case of transient high blood pressure. (For more on chronic high blood pressure, see the "Chronic high blood pressure" section earlier in this chapter.)

Transient high blood pressure is usually found for the first time after the middle of the pregnancy but without protein in the urine or any of the other signs or symptoms of preeclampsia. It doesn't cause any increased risk to the expectant mother or the fetus. Transient high blood pressure usually disappears a few days after delivery, but it's not entirely benign, however. It tends to occur again in future pregnancies, again not causing any problem, but it seems to be a marker for the development of essential high blood pressure (high blood pressure for which the cause is unknown) some years later.

Transient high blood pressure isn't treated during pregnancy because it seems to cause no setback for mother or fetus.

Dealing with High Blood Pressure after Delivery

After delivery has taken place, if the mother has chronic high blood pressure, three drugs can be used to manage the mother's high blood pressure while she breastfeeds. Methyldopa, timolol, and nifedipine (discussed in Chapter 13) can control high blood pressure. Although they're all excreted in breast milk, they haven't been found to hurt the baby in any way.

Discuss the possibility of withholding blood pressure medications while you breast-feed with your doctor. As long as you're carefully monitored for elevations in blood pressure, this can be done safely.

At this point, some of the other useful techniques for lowering blood pressure discussed in Part III can be safely added to the mother's program, especially salt reduction, weight loss, and exercise. Reducing salt, losing weight, and exercising speed up recovery from the stress of pregnancy and help to reduce blood pressure without the use of drugs.

Using Female Hormone Treatment in the Presence of High Blood Pressure

Women take estrogen and progesterone for two major indications, to prevent conception before menopause and to replace missing hormones after menopause. In the past, these hormones have been associated with increases in blood pressure. Current formulations of these medications aren't often associated with an increase in blood pressure, but it occasionally occurs. This section guides you through hormone use while avoiding the occurrence of high blood pressure.

Hormones for oral contraception

In the past, most women who took oral contraceptives were found to have a rise in blood pressure that was rarely severe and was usually mild. Just exactly how the oral contraceptives raise blood pressure is unknown. No particular factor, such as weight, age, or ethnic origin, seems to predict who will have an increase in blood pressure and to what extent. The newer preparations of oral contraceptives contain much smaller doses of both estrogen and progesterone. Increased blood pressure occurs less frequently with these preparations.

Women who smoke and are over age 35 are more sensitive to the oral contraceptives and shouldn't take them. The rise in blood pressure doesn't cause any damage to the body of most of these women, but occasionally, the kidneys are damaged. If concern exists about blood pressure, then discontinue the oral contraceptive.

If you plan to take oral contraceptives, you must stop smoking (which you should do even if you don't plan to take them). Make sure your blood pressure is measured before you start them and every 6 months while you take them. If you have a blood pressure increase of 20 mm Hg systolic or 10 mm Hg diastolic, you should stop the oral contraceptive in favor of a different form of contraception.

Drugs for increased blood pressure aren't usually given when oral contraceptives are believed to be the source of the increase, but occasionally no other form of contraception is possible. Then the usual treatment is used, beginning with lifestyle modification and using drugs to lower blood pressure if necessary.

Hormones for estrogen replacement

Because blood pressure rises as people age, some concern existed that estrogen replacement therapy would make this worse, given their known effect as part of the oral contraceptives. Estrogens are given in much lower doses for replacement therapy after menopause than the doses in oral contraceptives. Not only is estrogen replacement not a concern for high blood pressure, but the low dose of estrogen may actually lower blood pressure.

If a woman already has high blood pressure, estrogen therapy doesn't aggravate it. Estrogen replacement isn't used as treatment for high blood pressure, but the fact that it tends to lower blood pressure, if anything, means that it can be safely prescribed for the postmenopausal woman where blood pressure is a concern.

Part V
The Part of Tens

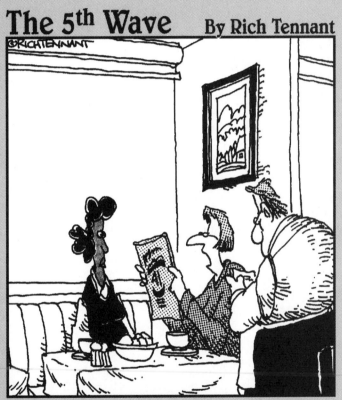

The 5th Wave   By Rich Tennant

"I'll have the 'Healthy-Heart-High-Fiber-Low-Fat-I'll-Just-Have-A-Bite-Of-My-Neighbor's-Eggs-Benedict Breakfast'."

In this part . . .

If you want to know simple tricks to lower your blood pressure and keep it normal, you can find them in this part. In addition, I provide a list of myths about treatment, so that you can avoid errors in treating your high blood pressure.

Discoveries about the topic of high blood pressure are being made all the time. In this part, you'll find some of these new discoveries. You'll also find some great resources for information that will inevitably be discovered after this book is marketed.

Chapter 17

Ten Simple Ways to Reduce Blood Pressure

In This Chapter

▶ Discovering tried-and-true ways to lower your blood pressure

▶ Incorporating pressure-lowering practices in your everyday life

Lowering your blood pressure and avoiding the organ damage that high blood pressure can cause isn't difficult. You can do so many things to lower your blood pressure: It's shocking that so many people are walking around with uncontrolled high blood pressure. Taking the suggestions in this chapter to heart and making them a priority in your everyday life can help lower your blood pressure and strengthen your heart — guaranteed.

You can consider your blood pressure to be under control if your measurement is 140/90 mm Hg or lower. For some people, especially people with diabetes, the number needs to be even lower. The lower you get your blood pressure, assuming you don't have dizziness, the better off you are. Don't smirk just because your blood pressure is 138/88 mm Hg. You would be better off with a blood pressure of 135/85 mm Hg — or even better, 130/80 mm Hg.

In this chapter, I offer ten of the many ways that you can lower your blood pressure. All of them are fairly simple. You actually know what you have to do already. Do I need to tell you to stop smoking and drinking? Do mice play baseball?

The trick is to adopt at least two of the ideas described in this chapter. If you succeed at both, you'll be well on your way to reducing your blood pressure to an agreeable level. If you succeed with one, you'll be on your way but may still need a boost, so try to tackle another tip. Most importantly, after you have made a change, keep at it! Don't fall back into old bad habits, or, if you do, consider it water under the bridge (or blood through the heart) and go on and make that change permanent. Now is the time to make a change. In the immortal words of Shakespeare in his play *Henry IV,* "Strike now, or else the iron cools."

Making Sure You Have High Blood Pressure

Most of the changes in this chapter are good for you whether you have high blood pressure or not. The exception is taking drugs. If you don't need drugs, don't take them. They come with side effects, and they're expensive. Trying to remember if you took them can drive you crazy as well as where you left them and wondering what they're doing for you. You don't need drugs if your blood pressure isn't high.

You may save yourself a lifetime of taking unnecessary drugs by making sure that your blood pressure truly is elevated, and remains elevated. Therefore, step one for reducing your blood pressure is to be certain that your blood pressure is persistently elevated. Blood pressure measurements can vary so that a single high reading is not acceptable for a diagnosis of high blood pressure. It should be confirmed with additional readings several weeks apart.

Make sure that your doctor is measuring your blood pressure properly. Numerous aspects of a blood pressure measurement can affect the accuracy of the reading: For example, the blood pressure cuff may be the wrong size; the arm may not be placed properly; you may not have had time to relax for a few minutes before the measurement; or you may have spoken during the measurement. (Tips for taking an accurate blood pressure measurement are covered in Chapter 2.)

In addition, make sure that you don't have *white coat high blood pressure,* blood pressure that's high only in the doctor's office when you may be nervous. Getting a good home blood pressure device is certainly worthwhile, so you can check your pressure at home. Having a blood pressure gauge at home may also be useful for following your response to treatment of any kind. Ask your doctor to recommend a reliable and inexpensive home device. Check it against your doctor's blood pressure measurement every six months or so to make sure that the device remains accurate.

If you take your own blood pressure, don't rely on a device in a pharmacy. The devices are notorious for their high error rate. Make sure the device is properly maintained before you rely on it.

Elevated blood pressure doesn't necessarily persist. You may have had some temporary reason for an elevation that disappears with time. If you're on medication, ask your doctor if you can lower the dose or even stop it if it's safe to do so after having taken it for a year or more. You may be able to avoid a lifetime of taking drugs.

Determining If You Have Secondary High Blood Pressure

As you know, most of the time, doctors don't know why you have high blood pressure. About 5 percent of the time, a definite treatable cause exists. In this case, high blood pressure is *secondary high blood pressure.* If doctors can discover a treatable cause for the high blood pressure, they can cure it, and you can lose your high blood pressure especially if it's found early enough. Because it's so unusual to find a curable form of high blood pressure, it's not advisable to put every patient with high blood pressure through numerous expensive tests looking for a needle in a haystack. If the haystack can be shrunk, however, it may be worthwhile. Doctors try to find clues that suggest your high blood pressure is secondary to another disease.

A patient is more likely to have secondary high blood pressure if her high blood pressure develops suddenly in childhood or past the age of 50 or if she is resistant to treatment with drugs. Changes in the shape and pigmentation of the body suggest that the high blood pressure is associated with another disease. If the patient is getting attacks of warmth and redness along with the high blood pressure, the patient should be examined thoroughly. Because high blood pressure tends to run in families, a person who doesn't have relatives with high blood pressure is more likely to have secondary high blood pressure.

When a suspicion of secondary high blood pressure exists, specific testing, as outlined in Chapter 4, is needed. Again, the shotgun approach isn't appropriate. Shooting at every diagnosis, hoping that one will hit the target, is wasteful and usually unproductive. The doctor should have a specific diagnosis in mind and then do the tests for that diagnosis.

Unfortunately, kidney damage is frequently the cause of secondary high blood pressure. Because the kidney can't be repaired at this point, the patient has to take blood pressure medication anyway. Knowing that the kidneys are already damaged is important, so the doctor can prescribe specific blood pressure drugs that are better for the kidneys. The doctor also knows that the kidney damage shouldn't be blamed on the high blood pressure.

If you have treatable secondary high blood pressure, you may be saved a lifetime of taking medication. If the primary disease is properly diagnosed and treated early, you may also be able to prevent the other damage that can be caused by it.

Giving Up Tobacco and Excess Alcohol

Both tobacco and alcohol raise blood pressure. Tobacco in any form, whether smoked, chewed, or snuffed does this. Drinking excessive amounts of alcohol, that is, more than two glasses of wine for a man or a glass of wine for a woman every night, raises blood pressure. Elevation of blood pressure is just the tip of the iceberg when it comes to the havoc that these addicting substances can wreak.

Smoking and drinking often go hand in hand. It may be better to concentrate on stopping one of them and, therefore, eliminating many of the situations where you do the other.

Terminating tobacco use

This is a no-brainer! I know how hard it is to stop smoking. You're addicted. But millions of people stop it in the United States every year. Believe me, they do not know something that you don't. You are part of a shrinking group, but you still make up 27 percent of the population if you smoke. That's about the same percent that has high blood pressure, although it's not the same 27 percent. These statistics come from the National Institutes of Health.

Cigarettes raise blood pressure. About 33 percent of the people with high blood pressure are smokers. It's the nicotine in tobacco that raises blood pressure.

Any regular exposure to tobacco is dangerous. If you smoke, you're not only damaging your own health, but you're compromising the health of your loved ones as well. Spouses and children of smokers have a much higher rate of lung disease, asthma, and cancer than the spouses and children of nonsmokers. That's no way to treat someone you love.

In that respect, this is one place where doctors ask you to do as they do, not as they say. You will hardly find a physician anywhere anymore who still smokes. Do you think that's a coincidence? Doctors are certain of the harm that tobacco can do. And that includes cigars and pipes. Any regular exposure to tobacco is dangerous. And it raises blood pressure.

Cutting back on cocktails

Excessive alcohol is bad for your blood pressure. Not only does the alcohol increase your blood pressure, but also the kilocalories in alcohol can add many kilocalories to your daily total. A glass of wine can be 125 kilocalories. If you drink three or four glasses, you're adding 375 to 500 kilocalories to your daily total. Plus, the state you'll be in as a result of that much alcohol doesn't lend itself to careful eating and salt restriction. You'll probably consume plenty of peanuts or potato chips with your wine.

Recent studies seem to indicate that a glass or two of red wine protects your heart from heart disease. Something in the skin of the red grape, which is mixed with liquid during the first part of the preparation of the wine, provides the healthful ingredient. Too much of a good thing is bad for you, however.

If you keep your alcohol intake in check, you can avoid abusing alcohol and raising your blood pressure. Men shouldn't drink more than two glasses of wine a day. Women shouldn't drink more than one glass of wine a day. If you prefer beer, two 12-ounce cans should be your limit if you're a male; one can of beer should be your limit if you're female. As for hard liquor, a man should consume no more than three ounces of distilled spirits, and a woman shouldn't consume more than one and a half ounces.

If you're a heavy drinker, try to decrease your intake gradually. Stopping abruptly can lead to a sudden rise in blood pressure. Check Chapter 11 for advice on how to stop drinking. If you believe you drink excessively, your intake should be zero ounces. Even a taste tends to get you started drinking excessively again.

Reducing Salt in Your Diet

So you do have high blood pressure after all, and you want to bring it under control because you're aware of the damage that it can do to your body. The easiest change that you can make is to take as much salt out of your diet as possible.

Don't worry that you won't get enough salt. You find salt in practically everything. Most Americans consume 5,000 milligrams (or three teaspoons) of salt each day. Yet they could get along quite well with only 500 milligrams (or one-third teaspoon). You'd achieve this desired amount if you only ate natural foods. However, although eating only 500 milligrams of salt a day is a great goal, lowering your intake to 1,500 milligrams a day is more realistic.

Prepared foods account for 75 percent of the salt in your diet. In an effort to reduce your salt intake, cut back on the number of prepared foods that you buy, such as prepared soups and crackers. Consult the Nutrition Facts label to check the amount of salt in each portion. Even if the salt content appears low, eating too many portions can put your salt level over the top. Start by cutting back on one of the biggest sources of salt in most diets: the chips and crackers that many people love to eat. You need to replace these snacks with low-salt chips or, even better, fresh fruit or raw vegetables.

Another 10 percent of the salt that you eat is found naturally in food, but the final 15 percent is what you add when you grab the saltshaker. Try keeping the saltshaker off the table.

Salt came into our diets in the first place when it was added to preserve food. Now that food is preserved with refrigeration and many other techniques, salt doesn't need to be added.

Many people don't like certain foods unless they're heavily salted. These saltaholics are missing all kinds of great tastes. If you fall into this category, try preparing your food with half the salt that you usually add. Tastes that you didn't know existed may pleasantly surprise you. You can finally experience the natural tastes of the food you eat when it's not overwhelmed by salt.

If you still need more flavor, though, try adding herbs and spices. You can find just about any variety at the supermarket. In many cases, you can add plain water to wash out much of the salt in canned vegetables and then adding herbs and spices to give the vegetables new tastes.

Eating out makes monitoring the amount of salt in your food rather difficult. Chefs tend to add salt liberally. When eating at a restaurant, ask for the food to be prepared with little or no salt or choose a restaurant that offers low-salt items on the menu. Your local branch of the American Heart Association often has a listing of local restaurants that serve low-salt food.

If your diet is heavy on the salt, you may be able to eliminate a drug that you're taking for high blood pressure by significantly reducing the salt. Tell me that's not a bargain!

Adopting the DASH Diet

A study published in the *New England Journal of Medicine* (April 1997) introduces the *Dietary Approach to Stop Hypertension* (DASH) diet. This diet, discussed in detail in Chapter 9, may be the best thing to come along for the treatment of high blood pressure in decades. Without having to cut kilocalories and depriving yourself, you can lower your blood pressure by the same amount as one of the good drugs for high blood pressure can.

The DASH diet requires you to eat a mix of grains, fruits, and vegetables and low-fat or nonfat dairy products while you reduce the intake of high-fat dairy products, meats, fats, and sweets. The diet also encourages a weekly ration of nuts and seeds. When the program is followed properly, the results are remarkable. People with the highest blood pressure seem to benefit the most.

One of the best features of the DASH diet is that the recommended foods are the ones you eat each day. No special supplements, vitamins, or minerals are needed. No daily visits to group therapy are required. You don't need to take a drug that reduces your appetite because you're not reducing your kilocalories. You aren't left feeling hungry. You don't even have to exercise in order to lower your pressure. (Although I urge you to do so.) After a while, you won't even miss all the meat and dairy products that fill your plate now. You're still getting some of that stuff anyway — just not so much.

People who adopt the DASH diet typically find that they can follow it permanently. This is unusual for most diets. You don't even have to change your diet all at once. Start reducing the meat and dairy and substituting some grains. Add more vegetables and use fruits for dessert instead of cookies, cake, or ice cream. Before you know it, you'll be DASHing. The effect on your blood pressure will be remarkable!

Combining DASH with a reduction in salt can double the lowering effects on your high blood pressure. If you follow the DASH diet, salt reduction takes place automatically. DASH contains foods that you usually prepare, rather than an outsider (such as a food manufacturer). Don't add salt to food and try to keep your salt intake under 1,500 milligrams every day.

Alternately, consider using the services of a knowledgeable dietitian. Make sure that he is well versed in the requirements of DASH. If you don't have a dietitian available to you, an excellent Web site that will answer most of your questions about the DASH diet, the appropriate foods, and the foods to avoid (after you read Chapter 9) is `www.nhlbi.nih.gov/hbp/prevent/h_eating/ h_eating.htm`.

Losing Weight by Reducing Kilocalorie Intake

A great way to lower your blood pressure is to lose weight. And the best way to lose weight is to reduce the number of kilocalories that you eat each day. You need to reduce your kilocalorie intake by 3,500 kilocalories to lose a pound of fat. (See Chapter 9 for more information on determining your daily caloric needs and deciding how much weight you need to lose to help lower your blood pressure.) You can do it by cutting out 500 kilocalories daily for a week or 250 kilocalories daily for two weeks or go even slower.

If you're overweight or obese with high blood pressure, you may want to really hit the jackpot: Combine DASH with low salt and weight loss. First, you might want to determine if you're overweight or obese. Take your weight in pounds, multiply it by 705, divide that result by your height in inches and divide that result by your height in inches again. If your result (called the body mass index BMI) is 25 to 29.9, then you are *overweight*. If the result is 30 or above, then you're *obese*. Use these numbers for convenience. You're not out of the woods if your BMI is 24.5. You'll still be better off with a BMI of 23.5 in terms of risking the complications from high blood pressure.

You really didn't need to do that calculation to know that you need to lose a few pounds, did you? Your pants are a little tighter, and your spouse recently made a remark about love handles. What are you going to do about it?

The key term here for reducing the number of kilocalories in your diet is *substitution*. Simply substitute a low-calorie food for a higher-calorie food. For example, instead of eating a handful of cookies, eat an apple. That substitution represents about 100 kilocalories saved. Combine that with a reduction in the size of your typical steak from 10 ounces to 3 ounces. That decrease in portion size represents a decrease of 800 kilocalories more or less. Do these kinds of substitutions for just four days, and you're a pound lighter.

Some of the best substitutions that you can make include:

- Adding your own fruit to plain yogurt instead of eating prepared fruit yogurt
- Snacking on fruits and vegetables rather than chips and soft drinks
- Drinking noncaloric soft drinks rather than sugary soft drinks
- Eating skinless white-meat chicken instead of dark-meat chicken with skin
- Choosing nonfat or low-fat dairy products in place of high-fat cheeses
- Using nonfat salad dressing rather than fatty salad dressings
- If selecting prepared food, choosing foods with fewer kilocalories instead of foods that have less fat

Use the Nutrition Facts label on all prepared foods to find out how much fat, kilocalories, and salt you'll be taking in if you eat a portion of any food. As a careful observer of supermarket shoppers, I rarely see anyone looking at the label. The government has gone to so much trouble to get the food producers to label their foods. Give them a look.

Food preparation is key because it's a point where many kilocalories can be added to food or where kilocalories can be cut back, depending on the method used. Foods that are broiled, cooked in their own juices, poached, grilled, blackened, or baked are preferred, whether you're cooking for yourself or eating in a restaurant. Those foods that are battered and fried or made in a butter, cream, plum, cheese, or sweet-and-sour sauce should be avoided.

Losing weight and keeping it off can be difficult, but you can definitely do it. The key to success is the level of your motivation. If joining a weight-loss group helps keep you motivated, do it. People often do well in a group setting but slip back when they're on their own. I urge my patients to continue contact with whatever weight-loss group they belong to. Every study I have seen shows the value of continuing to participate on a regular basis. Check out the "Characteristics of successful losers" sidebar in Chapter 9. The bottom line is that these individuals tried to lose weight multiple times, but they finally succeeded when they ate fewer kilocalories and exercised regularly.

Starting an Exercise Program

If you don't want to lose weight or curb your salt intake (although I strongly advise both), you can still lower your blood pressure with exercise. But you have to choose an exercise program that you can stick to. Too many people start their exercise around January 1 each year and end it on January 15. They're New Year's Resolution exercisers. Their plan requires much more than they're prepared to do on a long-term basis, so the regimen doesn't last.

To start your exercise program, make sure you're in good enough health to take on the exercise you plan to do. A visit to the doctor for a checkup can take care of that.

Make up a program that starts slow for short distances and builds up until you're doing 45 minutes of exercise three or four times a week. This sounds like a walking or jogging program, and that's what I think works best for most people. You don't have to join a club to do it. How often do you see someone take an elevator up to a health club to go on the StairMaster? Check Chapter 12 for a complete program for walking and jogging.

A walking or jogging program is certainly an attainable goal, but you still have to make yourself do it. Don't make excuses. Some of my patients tell me that they're too tired to exercise when they get home after working. This stands to reason. They *are* tired — because they're in bad shape from lack of exercise (unless their work consists of manual labor). The problem arises when these patients, continuing the vicious cycle, decide not to exercise. So put on those sneakers, and start moving!

Exercising after work may not be the best option for you, especially if you have kids or work late hours. If you find that evenings don't work for you, try exercising in the morning or during your lunch break. Finding a time that works for you helps to prevent you from skipping your workouts.

You may be one of those people who just can't get motivated on their own. If so, choose a competitive sport that you can do regularly. A partner will be waiting for you, so you can't make excuses. Tennis is a great choice, but weather often limits the times that you can play, unless you go to an indoor court. You'd probably be better off doing *some* tennis, *some* jogging, and *some* swimming rather than sticking to only one. This variation of activity is called *cross-training.* Besides the fact that cross-training allows you to have something to do whatever the weather, this kind of program may be more interesting in the long run (pun intended). Cross-training also tones a wider range of muscle groups.

Another form of exercise that you may want to add to your cross-training is weight lifting. Don't start lifting megatons at the beginning. Start off lifting a light weight and work your way up slowly. *Note:* If you have stage 3 high blood pressure (greater than 180/110 mm Hg), weight lifting isn't a good idea, but everyone else at lower levels of high blood pressure can benefit from it. Don't forget to warm up and cool down. You perform much better if you warm up before you exercise, and give your body a chance to gradually return to a quiet state if you slow the pace for a while before stopping.

And be sure to use the right equipment. Buying a more expensive pair of running shoes is worth every penny when you consider how those shoes can protect the cartilage in your knees.

Exercise doesn't just lower blood pressure. It increases self-esteem, improves balance, fights depression, enhances memory, and generally makes you very aware that life is worth living.

If you're overweight and have been diagnosed with high blood pressure, you can hit the jackpot if you adopt the DASH diet (Chapter 9), reduce your salt intake (Chapter 10), reduce your kilocalorie intake (Chapter 9 and 12), and exercise (Chapter 12). Besides, you'll be healthier, thinner, and have lower blood pressure all at once!

Enhancing Your Treatment with Mind-Body Techniques

Some disciplines that are associated with Eastern philosophies lower blood pressure. I'm not suggesting that you should ignore Western medicine and follow the paths of the East; however, using mind-body techniques, such as yoga, meditation, and hypnosis, can enhance your current course of treatment. If you can get a few millimeters of mercury of blood pressure down with one or several mind-body practices, it's worthwhile — not to mention the other benefits you can get of out it, such as a focused and serene mind. (See Chapter 12 for more information on mind-body techniques.)

Mind-body techniques should be an *addition* to the salt reduction, weight loss, and exercise that you do already, not a substitute — something that you engage in to take the place of the medications that you're taking. Don't stop these on your own. Work with your doctor every step of the way. If you receive a suggestion from a friend or read about a technique that strikes your fancy, by all means, try it. After you become proficient, you can think about stopping a blood pressure medication under the supervision of your doctor.

I limited myself to a discussion of these four — yoga, meditation, hypnosis, and biofeedback — but human beings have a way of controlling every function in the body. One of my favorites is humor therapy. (See Chapter 8 for more on humor therapy.) If you walk into a room where everyone is laughing for no apparent reason, you may have found your way into a humor club. Imagine! They don't even need a source of humor. They just go ahead and laugh, regardless of the consequences, which may include a fall in blood pressure. In addition to lowering blood pressure, laughter can also reduce stress hormones and improve immune function. Try it, you'll like it.

Yoga

Yoga is older than the other mind-body practices and seems to be experiencing a major revival. It emphasizes postures and proper breathing. People coming out of a yoga class almost always relate how relaxed and warm they feel. When their blood pressure is taken, it's usually lower than before the class. Every health club seems to have a few yoga classes, and more and more yoga institutes are opening in various areas. The quality of the teaching seems to remain at a high level, despite the tremendous increase in the resources available.

Meditation

Meditation is a technique for calming the mind by concentrating on an object, a sound, a word, or the breath. Just as it calms the mind, meditation appears to calm the blood pressure as well. You don't have to spend hours a day sitting quietly, either. Just a few minutes of meditation each day seems to be enough to provide a day's worth of blood pressure control. For those of you who are against exercise in any form, this method of sitting quietly may be just the blood pressure-lowering technique you've been looking for.

Hypnosis

If you want something even more passive than meditation, try hypnosis. You can hypnotize yourself. By the process of self-suggestion, you can tell yourself to be calm and to lower your stress level and your blood pressure. If you need help figuring out how to hypnotize yourself, many resources are available on the Internet. (For some Web site suggestions, see Chapter 12.) Hypnotism isn't a "game," but a useful tool that may be your answer to controlling your blood pressure.

Biofeedback

Biofeedback is a technique for training oneself with the aid of *biofeedback machines* that detect a person's internal bodily functions (such as high blood pressure), so that the functions can be altered. You control the output of the machine (such as a flashing light) by relaxing your muscles. As your muscles relax, your tension and your blood pressure fall. After you've developed control over your body tension with a machine, you can do it without the machine. Because biofeedback requires equipment, it may be a little less desirable than the other methods. But if you can't engage in the other mind-body techniques for some reason, then this may be the solution for you.

Using Drugs to Lower Blood Pressure

You've tried every technique short of medication, and you still see more than 140/90 mm Hg when you check your blood pressure. First of all, don't blame yourself unless you know that you could've done much better. If that's the case, go back and try working on your diet, salt intake, and exercise program again. If you think that you've given drug-free forms of treatment a run for their money, however, and haven't received the desired result, you need to discuss blood pressure medication options with your doctor. More than 60 different medications are available for lowering blood pressure, so you're sure to find the right drug or combination of drugs for your needs. Even though more than 60 are available, most people use the same three types, which also happen to be the least expensive and most-known by doctors. Most people do just fine with just one, two, or three medications — alone or in combination. (For more information on blood-pressure-lowering drugs, see Chapter 13.)

Not taking the prescription pills that you have in your possession is what we doctors call *noncompliance* — a major crime if ever there was one. Noncompliance doesn't do much for your blood pressure.

More than likely, your doctor will start you out with a *diuretic* (a medication that lowers blood pressure by forcing the body to rid itself of salt and water through the kidneys into the urine). Hydrochlorothiazide is as effective as any of them, and it's available as a generic. Unfortunately, the dosage that has been shown to be most effective, both for lowering blood pressure and prolonging life, is not yet manufactured. So you have to buy the 25-milligram (mg) pill and break it in half to get the 12.5-mg dose. And that, with a little bit of luck, may be all that you need. If you're already on a bigger dose, see if you can talk your doctor into reducing it while monitoring your blood pressure. He may be surprised, but you won't be because you've read this book.

If the diuretic doesn't do the job or you want to get your blood pressure down even lower because you're diabetic, ask your doctor about adding a *beta blocker* (a medication that blocks pressure-raising substances in the body). The beta blocker propranolol, probably the best of the beta blockers for treatment of high blood pressure, has also been around for decades and has proven itself.

One problem with the beta blockers is that they can cause fatigue and reduce exercise tolerance. Subsequently, beta blockers aren't a good choice for people who do strenuous exercise. Propranolol is probably the best of the beta blockers for treatment of high blood pressure.

If diuretics and beta blockers don't control your high blood pressure completely, your doctor may prescribe a *calcium channel blocking agent* (a medication that widens blood vessels). By themselves, they're not as effective as diuretics or beta blockers, but together they may do the job. They're a poor choice as the first drug to be used, especially if any heart failure is present or a heart attack has already occurred. Beta blockers are much more valuable in that situation. If your doctor suggests taking a calcium channel blocker, ask if Nifedipine Extended-release Tablets may work for you. It's inexpensive because it's a generic pill, and it only needs to be taken once a day.

Finally, for the purposes of my brief discussion in this section, one of the drugs from the class called *angiotensin-converting enzyme* (ACE) *inhibitors* or the similar class called *angiotensin II receptor blockers* may need to be added. You'd probably not want to take four different drugs for high blood pressure. Add this to the diuretic and the beta blocker for a three-drug combination, if needed. Of course, for some people, especially diabetics with kidney disease,

ACE inhibitors and angiotensin II receptor blockers are the treatment of choice because they not only lower blood pressure but also protect the kidneys. Of the many drugs in these classes, enalapril or lisinopril are once-a-day and inexpensive. Don't take these two types of drugs during a pregnancy or while breastfeeding. They're not good for the baby.

I thoroughly discuss many other drugs in Chapter 13, but they have limited use for controlling high blood pressure with the possible exception of methyldopa, the favorite drug of obstetricians for their pregnant women with high blood pressure. If your doctor prescribes one of the other drugs, you can find more information about it in Chapter 13.

With all the blood pressure drugs available, one is certain to work for you. There's absolutely no excuse for not controlling blood pressure, preventing heart attacks, brain attacks, and kidney damage. And yet only 12.5 million of the 50 million people with high blood pressure in the United States are under control. Let's improve that statistic one patient at a time — starting with you or your loved one.

Avoiding Drugs That Raise Blood Pressure

Plenty of drugs are on the market that actually *raise* blood pressure on their own or because they block the action of a drug that lowers blood pressure. If you can possibly avoid them, do so. Sometimes, however, the problem that makes you need the other drug is so severe that you can't avoid it. You then have to use the drugs for high blood pressure to overcome the blood pressure elevation of the essential drug.

Monitor your blood pressure whenever you start or stop a drug. The new drug may raise the blood pressure or block your own blood pressure drugs. A drug that you were taking and are now stopping may also have interacted with your blood pressure medication in some way, so that your pressure was under control when you used the drug but will rise when you stop it.

Many cold medications contain drugs that cause constriction of arteries and elevation of blood pressure. You need to read the label on any cold medication that you plan to use. The label should say clearly that it contains medications that should not be taken by a person who has high blood pressure. If uncertain, check with your doctor before you use it.

Certain diet pills contain phenylpropa-nolamine. This drug, which is similar to amphetamine, raises blood pressure. You shouldn't use these drugs if you have high blood pressure already. Yet millions of people take them to slim down.

Of the drugs that your doctor may prescribe for you, many steroids, such as cortisone or prednisone, raise blood pressure. Several of the antidepressant drugs, particularly trimipramine and venlafaxine, have caused sustained increases in blood pressure. Other antidepressant drugs from the class called *monoamine oxidase inhibitors* raise blood pressure by preventing the breakdown of epinephrine. Drugs in this class include phenylzine and tranylcypromine. Any of the nonsteroidal anti-inflammatory agents also raise blood pressure. The worst offenders are indomethacin, naprosyn, and ibuprofen, especially in large doses.

Certain drugs that fight against your blood pressure medications make your blood pressure medication less effective. Numerous drugs fall into this category, some of which you can't avoid if you have certain problems. For example, if you have kidney disease, you may have to take erythropoietin to combat anemia. As much as you don't need another way for your blood pressure to elevate, erythropoietin will do it. But you have to take it because it's the only way to increase your blood count — besides transfusions, which don't tend to keep your count higher for very long.

Colestipol, a drug for lowering cholesterol, is another one that fights against blood pressure medications. Fortunately, the choices for treating cholesterol are numerous, so this drug can be stopped, if necessary. Cholestyramine is also a cholesterol-lowering drug with the same tendency to raise blood pressure.

Oral contraceptives, when they contained higher amounts of estrogen, were notorious for raising blood pressure. The newer preparations with less estrogen are much better in that respect. You still should have your blood pressure checked before you start taking an oral contraceptive and have it checked every so often after you're on them. Estrogen taken for menopause, however, may actually lower blood pressure.

Some antacids contain an abundance of salt, which you know doesn't help your blood pressure. Check the label before you decide to buy a particular antacid. If you're taking in 900 milligrams of salt each time your stomach aches, you aren't doing your blood pressure any favors. You can find plenty of good choices, such as various calcium-containing antacids and magnesium-containing antacids, so read the label to see what you're getting!

Illegal drugs that raise blood pressure, such as cocaine, shouldn't be taken in the first place, much less by a person who has high blood pressure.

I've only given you a partial list. Some drugs may raise blood pressure in only one person — you! Check with your doctor to make sure that your new medication doesn't raise your blood pressure or block your blood pressure drugs.

Chapter 18

Ten Myths About High Blood Pressure

● ●

In This Chapter

▶ Investigating misunderstandings about high blood pressure

▶ Discovering the realities of high blood pressure

● ●

*M*yths about high blood pressure are numerous, and selecting only ten is difficult. I tried to pick out the myths that have the most impact on your high blood pressure. People are likely to believe myths when they don't have an understanding of a subject. Myths often provide a justification for a certain action or inaction. It's my hope that after you have your misunderstandings cleared up by this chapter, you'll take many or all of the actions described in Part III and take complete control of your blood pressure. Taking control of your blood pressure can help you avoid the medical consequences described in Part II.

Feeling Fine and Skipping Blood Pressure Medications

High blood pressure is sometimes called the "silent killer." People are often unaware that they have high blood pressure. It can do damage to the eyes, heart, kidneys, and blood vessels, but symptoms don't appear until an organ begins to fail. When the organ begins to fail, it's too late to reverse the damage.

A lack of symptoms is the reason that many people neglect to take their blood pressure medication. They felt fine before they started taking the pills. The only reason they're taking the pills is because their doctor measured a high blood pressure. In fact, as a result of the side effects of the pills, they may feel worse when taking the pills.

Not taking your blood pressure medication isn't a good idea. The point of taking the medication is to lower your pressure and in turn, to prevent complications, such as heart attacks and brain attacks (described in Part II). These complications probably take ten years or more to develop. Bringing your blood pressure down into the normal range through lifestyle changes and medication if necessary gives you time to steer clear of these complications.

If side effects from the medication are a problem, discuss the possibility of lowering the dose or switching to another medicine with your doctor.

Medications can help you control your blood pressure and avoid the serious damage, or even death, that high blood pressure causes. Don't fail to make use of them.

Needing Treatment Only for a High Diastolic Blood Pressure

Treating a high diastolic blood pressure only was once the way that blood pressure control was practiced, and it hasn't disappeared from the treatment plan of many doctors. But you know better.

Both the diastolic blood pressure and the systolic blood pressure figure in the decision to lower blood pressure. The goal is to maintain a number under 140 for the systolic blood pressure and a number under 90 for the diastolic blood pressure.

Diastolic blood pressure tends to fall with age while systolic blood pressure tends to rise. For example, studies show that people under the age of 50 who have high blood pressure usually have diastolic high blood pressure. The much larger group of people over the age of 50 who have high blood pressure usually has isolated systolic high blood pressure. According to these numbers, if treatment were based on the diastolic blood pressure alone, very few people would receive treatment for high blood pressure detected after the age of 50. Yet treating people over age 50 for high blood pressure greatly reduces the number of heart attacks and brain attacks in this age group.

Studies also show that systolic high blood pressure can predict whether people over 50 are likely to develop coronary atherosclerosis (see Chapter 5).

In the group under 50, diastolic high blood pressure was most predictive of coronary atherosclerosis. But in the group over 50, systolic high blood pressure was a better predictor of coronary atherosclerosis.

At the same time, it should be noted that lowering the diastolic blood pressure too much in the elderly population (older than 75) is dangerous. Because their diastolic blood pressure is already low, reducing it below 65 to 70 mm Hg with blood pressure medication results in an increase of brain attacks. In this case, accepting a systolic blood pressure greater than 140 may be necessary in order to avoid a diastolic blood pressure below 70.

Thinking High Blood Pressure Can't Be Controlled

If you're diagnosed with high blood pressure and take your medication regularly, but your blood pressure doesn't come down into the acceptable range of 140/90 mm Hg, don't give up — and definitely don't stop taking your medication. Instead, with the help of your doctor, take another look a your medication and lifestyle to see if you can do more to control your blood pressure. Rest assured, an explanation for your inability to bring your blood pressure under control can be found. The means to control high blood pressure in all patients currently exist. It's up to you and your doctor to find the right solution.

Start by making sure that your blood pressure is uncontrolled. Could it be a case of faulty measurement? Is your blood pressure normal except when you step into the doctor's office (white coat effect)? You may have to get your own blood pressure device and check it for yourself at home.

Take a closer look at your medication. Resistance to treatment is defined as the inability of a combination of three different types of medications from three different classes, one of which is a diuretic, to lower the blood pressure to less than 140/90 mm Hg. Is it possible that you have low potassium as a result of too much diuretic? Are you an African American taking a beta blocker, which lowers blood pressure less effectively among African Americans? Are you taking one daily dose of a medication that doesn't last through a full 24 hours? Maybe you're currently treating another medical problem with medications that are interfering with the action of your blood pressure medicines? Check with your doctor to see if any drug interactions are blocking your blood pressure treatment.

Are you maximizing your use of lifestyle changes to squeeze every millimeter of mercury out of those procedures? Are you reducing your salt intake? Have you lost some weight and kept it off? It doesn't take much — only 5 to 10 percent of your body weight — to make a big dent in your blood pressure. Have you tried the DASH diet (described in Chapter 9), which in many cases can lower your blood pressure as much as the best blood pressure medications? Have you quit smoking? Have you reduced or stopped your intake of caffeine? Have you stopped drinking more than a glass or two of wine daily? Are you trying some of the other methods, such as yoga, meditation, or laughter? You can't say that your blood pressure can't be controlled until all these methods have been put to use.

Next, discuss the possibility that you have secondary high blood pressure (see Chapter 4) with your doctor. The diseases and conditions that can cause second high blood pressure, such as blocked kidney arteries or a tumor in an adrenal gland, are rare but may account for the stubborn resistance of your blood pressure to treatment.

Believing the Treatment is Worse Than the Disease

The consequences of untreated high blood pressure at any age are far greater than the side effects of medication or the inconveniences of lifestyle changes. To begin with, use nondrug treatments, such as lowering your salt and caffeine intake and exercising regularly, to their fullest extent. (See Chapters 8 through 12 for more ways that you can adjust your lifestyle to lower your blood pressure.) Many of the nondrug treatments not only lower your blood pressure but also provide you with all kinds of other benefits. The peacefulness that comes from exercising, yoga, and meditation can't be found in any blood pressure medicine.

If your doctor determines that your blood pressure should be treated with medication, don't have a crisis. Sure, blood pressure medications have side effects, and you'll probably feel better without them. But there aren't too many side effects that are worse than the effects of untreated high blood pressure — namely heart attacks, brain attacks, and kidney failure.

The side effects can be overcome in several ways. Ask your doctor if you can lower your dose of medication while monitoring your blood pressure. If the side effects are severe, ask your doctor to prescribe two different medications at lower doses to avoid the side effects of either. If you're fatigued, ask your doctor to check your potassium and add a potassium-sparing agent (see Chapter 13) if it's low. A number of blood pressure medications cause sleepiness. If you perform some work that requires high mental alertness, such as running heavy equipment or driving a car, let your doctor know, because these drugs are probably not the ones for you. Work with your doctor to determine the combination of lifestyle changes and medications that's right for you.

If you're a competitive athlete, the beta blockers are probably a poor choice for you because they prevent your body from changing its heart rate and other parameters that are necessary for vigorous activity. Certain drugs, such as angiotensin-converting enzyme (ACE) inhibitors, are especially helpful under special circumstances, such as diabetic kidney disease. You wouldn't want to lose the great benefits of these drugs because you refuse to take drugs.

Limiting the Treatment to Nervous, Anxious People

A high level of nervousness and anxiety doesn't indicate that a person has or will have high blood pressure. A nervous, anxious person may have normal blood pressure, while a person who appears quite calm and peaceful may have exceedingly high blood pressure.

This myth probably developed from the short name for high blood pressure — hypertension. The prefix *hyper* suggests that sufferers are highly stressed, jumpy, and nervous individuals, who live a life of anger and road rage and have a short fuse, making them ready to blow up at any moment. The suffix *tension* certainly doesn't suggest a calm, peaceful state of being. However, that people with high blood pressure come only from this group isn't the case.

People with high blood pressure are found in every social class, doing every type of work. And although high blood pressure tends to be a disease of the overweight, it's certainly found among thin people. People with high blood pressure aren't necessarily type A overachievers working 14 hour days. It would certainly make doctors' diagnostic abilities much better if they could pick out people who have high blood pressure from one group with certain personality traits, but it doesn't work that way.

It's true that acute stress raises the blood pressure temporarily. This is a normal body response to stress: Blood pressure rises in response to stress and the release of hormones. However, as stress becomes *chronic,* or lasts over a long period of time, the hormones are no longer released at the same rate, and the blood pressure falls.

People who move from a quiet neighborhood to a big city are found to have an increase in blood pressure. But this is more the result of increased salt and weight gain than the stresses of the big city. Similarly, a stressful job raises the blood pressure temporarily in some people, especially men. But high blood pressure doesn't persist from the stress alone.

Avoiding Exercise Because of High Blood Pressure

This myth provides an excuse for many people who don't want to exercise. Not only is it totally and unequivocally false, but also the opposite is actually true. Exercise lowers blood pressure.

How did this myth get started? It may have begun in a dark alley in the Kasbah (just joking). Actually, it probably began when some people with severe, uncontrolled high blood pressure and major complications of the condition did some exercise and got into trouble. If you have unstable heart disease associated with high blood pressure, for example, you can have a heart attack as a result of heavy exercise.

If you have heart disease or if you have had a heart attack or a brain attack, ask your physician what exercises you can do safely. You may find that there are no limitations. Or you may find that it's safer for you to avoid certain activities that are too vigorous or require too much effort over a short period of time, such as heavy weight lifting. But there is no reason for you to avoid physical activity if your high blood pressure is under control. Many private doctors are unaware of how much you should do and will tell you to "take it easy." You need better advice than that, and you may want to see a cardiologist or an exercise physiologist.

If you have high blood pressure and no complications, the benefits of exercise are enormous. See the long list of exercises in Chapter 12. You don't have to run marathons or do triathlons. One half hour of walking a day provides great benefits. Select an exercise that you know you'll continue to do. There is no point in choosing sprinting because you can't do it for very long each time, and you won't want to keep doing it. You may want to choose an exercise that can be done indoors for those days of inclement weather. (Although I recently met a fanatic young woman who runs daily. When it rains, she uses a plastic garbage bag to keep dry.)

Don't feel that you have to push your limitations. Exercise that you perceive as "very hard" is about what you want to do. Some days you may want to do less. Don't exercise to the point that you have chest pain or can't breathe. Should that happen, you might want to confer with your doctor.

The old adage for physical exercise used to be, "No pain, no gain." The new one is, "Refrain, no gain."

Passing Up Treating the Elderly

Some people believe that it's too late or not helpful to treat high blood pressure in the elderly. High blood pressure is most prevalent in the elderly population, the people that I have arbitrarily selected as age 75 or older. They're also the people who have the highest number of heart attacks and brain attacks each year. If they get treatment for their high blood pressure, large numbers of these attacks can be prevented. If they're not treated, some of them die earlier than they might normally have, and some of them will be subjected to years of disability.

Treating the elderly is not a simple matter — that's why I devoted Chapter 14 to this subject. Just like children, they can't simply be left to care for themselves without supervision, unless it has been shown that they can do so.

The elderly usually show isolated systolic high blood pressure and low diastolic pressure. Great care must be taken not to lower the diastolic blood pressure too much — readings shouldn't be any lower than 60 to 70.

The elderly are especially sensitive to salt, which can raise blood pressure. Reducing the amount of salt in an elderly person's diet may successfully control their blood pressure. Because they have reduced taste sensation, they may want to add more salt than usual to their food. They can be taught to substitute herbs and spices for salt.

Lifestyle changes are preferable to drugs when it comes to the elderly. The elderly take an average of seven drugs each day, so avoiding additional drugs is a good idea.

The elderly have diminished kidney function, even when they have no diseases. If drugs are used to treat the elderly, they should be prescribed at the lowest initial doses possible and increased very slowly. The recommendation is to start low and go slow when treating elderly people with high blood pressure.

Restricting Your Life Because You Have High Blood Pressure

Although high blood pressure is a serious condition that must be managed with lifestyle change and drugs if necessary, restricting your life isn't reasonable. You should be able to live a normal life within the limitations of any side effects caused by the drugs that you're taking.

If you have uncomplicated high blood pressure, you should have about the same quality of life as a person with normal blood pressure. Your quality of life can be even better because you're taking better care of your body. You may consider limiting salt intake and kilocalories as a restriction on your life and to some extent they are. On the other hand, they could be looked upon as enhancing the quality of your life. Taking salt out of your diet gives you a chance to taste some amazing foods that were hidden behind the strong taste of salt. Restricting kilocalories and losing some weight makes you feel better about yourself, more attractive, and healthier.

If you must take a drug that makes you sleepy, you shouldn't work in a profession that requires maximum alertness. Other than that, there is no limitation to what you can do with your life, high blood pressure or not. I haven't seen any case where a person has been refused a job because of high blood pressure. In fact, in cases where a person has lost a job because of high blood pressure, the courts have ruled in favor of the employee. It's wrong to terminate an employee because of high blood pressure.

Giving Up Treatment of High Blood Pressure After a Heart or Brain Attack

You shouldn't stop treating high blood pressure after you recover from a heart or brain attack. The risks of complications from high blood pressure are great after a heart or brain attack; therefore, controlling your blood pressure after one of these attacks is important. One of the main risk factors for a heart attack or a brain attack is a previous heart or brain attack. You need to make sure that your blood pressure is kept under control more than ever.

Before you leave the hospital, you should be planning to make the changes that will bring your blood pressure under control. You want to stop smoking and follow a low-salt DASH diet (described in Chapter 9). You want to start a lifelong exercise program after your doctor has cleared you. You also want to reduce your alcohol intake if it's excessive.

The changes that you make to control your high blood pressure can help your diabetes and your arthritis, as well as your heart and blood vessels.

Assuming High Blood Pressure is Less Dangerous in Women

The consequences of high blood pressure for women are as serious as those for men. Blood pressure control is just as important for women as it is for men.

Although three out of four women who have high blood pressure are aware of it, only one of those three has the high blood pressure under control. In other words, 75 percent of women with high blood pressure don't control it. This is a tragic situation for many women with high blood pressure.

The extremely dangerous disorders called *preeclampsia* and *eclampsia* that can begin in the 20th week of a pregnancy are ignored only at great risk to the mother and the growing fetus (see Chapter 16).

Estrogen may play an important role in women who are postmenopausal with high blood pressure. Estrogen replacement therapy can lower blood pressure in these women by as much as 10/5 mm Hg.

Even at the other end of the age spectrum, women in their 70s and 80s represent a large proportion of the high blood pressure among all people at that age. Fifty percent of all white women and 80 percent of all black women in the United States over age 60 have high blood pressure. These women suffer heart attacks and brain attacks at a much higher rate when their high blood pressure isn't controlled.

Chapter 19

Ten New Discoveries About High Blood Pressure

*W*hen I went to the Internet site of the National Library of Medicine and typed in the words *high blood pressure* in the subject box, limiting the search to articles published from 1/1/2000 to 2/8/2002, I was offered 10,399 citations to browse. This number represents the articles on this subject that the National Library of Medicine catalogued from all the medical and scientific journals in the world. When I changed the search term to *hypertension,* the search brought up 17,121 separate publications.

The great number of articles published in a little over two years indicates the enormous amount of research going on to help doctors and patients understand and treat high blood pressure. Perhaps one of these publications can solve the problem and its complications, and a cure for high blood pressure is just around the corner. But until then, you can benefit from the discoveries of thousands of people around the world making their contribution to understanding high blood pressure. This chapter provides ten new discoveries related to the treating high blood pressure — a small sample of the published work on high blood pressure.

You can also check the literature for yourself. It's simple and free. Just go to the National Center for Biotechnology Information Web site: `www.ncbi.nlm.nih.gov/entrez/query.fcgi`, fill in the box that asks what you're searching for with the words *high blood pressure* or *hypertension* and be prepared to spend the next few days reading.

These articles were probably submitted for publication at least six months before they were published, and the research that they're based on took place a year or more before that. A lag exists between research and publication that's inevitable (and essential) so that scientists and researchers can review and check the information before it reaches the public.

Taking Medication

A University of Michigan study in the *Annals of Pharmacotherapy* (January 2002) looked for the reasons that some people took their medications for high blood pressure and others didn't. Out of the 102 patients studied, 68 percent took their medications routinely. The participants who did *not* take their medications regularly didn't bother to measure their blood pressure, but they believed that their blood pressure was under control (less than 140/90 mm Hg).

People with high blood pressure want to control it without the help of prescribed medications. However, rather than using objective high blood pressure measurements, they often use their own subjective feeling to determine whether their blood pressure is under control. Because high blood pressure is generally without symptoms, they're really unaware of whether their high blood pressure has been lowered.

You can't tell the level of your own blood pressure without a blood pressure measuring device. Do *not* use your subjective sense of your blood pressure as a reason to stop high blood pressure medication.

Recognizing the White Coat Effect

A visit to the doctor's office may be another factor that often causes a rise in blood pressure called the *white coat effect*. Without even trying, doctors (who often wear white lab coats) make patients feel uneasy because, when experiencing the white coat effect, a patient's systolic blood pressure may be several millimeters of mercury higher than when taken at home. Even the nurse can cause a white coat effect.

In the *Journal of Cardiology* (January 2002), a group from Japan attempted to evaluate the importance of the white coat effect on high blood pressure: Is it as significant as sustained high blood pressure, which is present all the time? The study looked at the occurrence of brain attacks, also called strokes (see Chapter 7), in 147 older Japanese with no high blood pressure as compared to 236 with white coat high blood pressure and 575 with sustained high blood pressure.

The study concluded that the incidence of brain attacks in older Japanese people with high blood pressure as a result of the white coat effect is similar to that of people without high blood pressure. But the likelihood of a brain attack among those with sustained high blood pressure is far greater. That is, high blood pressure from the white coat effect and no high blood pressure are about the same in predicting a future brain attack while sustained high blood pressure is at least four times as dangerous.

In the *American Journal of Hypertension* (December 2001), another important study of the white coat effect and high blood pressure suggested that so-called *resistant high blood pressure* (blood pressure that does not respond to drug treatment) is actually high blood pressure from the white coat effect, and it may not be resistant at all.

The study indicated that out of 611 patients with high blood pressure, 118 were taking at least three drugs in combination, but their blood pressure wasn't any lower than 135/85 mm Hg. All these patients were studied with 24-hour *ambulatory blood pressure monitoring* — an ambulatory blood pressure meter is worn that takes the blood pressure every five to ten minutes during the day and night. The study found that one-fourth of the incidence of high blood pressure thought to have been resistant was actually brought under control away from the doctor's office. It was only when the doctor or the nurse took the blood pressure that it was elevated. The study recommended that white coat high blood pressure be considered before a person is diagnosed as having resistant high blood pressure.

If your doctor thinks that your blood pressure is resistant to treatment, ask him to look at your blood pressure for a 24-hour period with an ambulatory blood-pressure monitoring device before doing any other investigation. Your high blood pressure may be under control after all.

Using Fixed-Dose Combinations of Medications

If your blood pressure can be controlled with a single drug, like a thiazide diuretic (described in Chapter 13), that's preferred. However, a second drug usually needs to be added in order to reach the blood pressure goal.

An article from the Medical College of Virginia in *Drugs* (March 2002) sings the praises of fixed-dose combinations and urges that they be made inexpensive so that these useful combinations can be taken full advantage of.

For many years, it has been possible to give a single pill that contains drugs from two different classes, but there has been a reluctance to use them. The mechanism in each drug lowers blood pressure, and the combination, besides the advantage of taking a single pill, reduces the amount of either drug that needs to be taken. In addition, one drug often counteracts the bad side effects of the other.

One combination that's been useful is a diuretic and a beta-adrenergic receptor blocker (see Chapter 13). The diuretic reverses the tendency of the beta blocker to cause salt and water retention. Another good combination is a calcium channel blocking agent with an angiotensin-converting enzyme (ACE) inhibitor (also described in Chapter 13). The calcium channel blocking agent often causes water retention and swelling of the legs while the ACE inhibitor tends to reverse this side effect. Diuretics may cause salt and water loss that results in the body producing too much aldosterone to overcome this. The aldosterone then causes potassium loss. This can be overcome with the use of an ACE inhibitor or an angiotensin II receptor blocker at the same time. Alternately, a potassium-sparing diuretic may be prescribed.

If a single drug is causing you problems because of side effects, ask your doctor if you can be placed on a fixed-dose combination, which may provide the benefits of both drugs in a convenient form while reducing the dose needed for either.

Treating High Blood Pressure in Diabetics

When a patient has both diabetes and high blood pressure, the danger of complications of either disease is much greater. Diabetes tends to affect the eyes, the kidneys, and the nervous system as well as the heart. Similarly, high blood pressure tends to affect the heart and the kidneys and can damage the eyes and blood vessels as well.

The goal for treating high blood pressure when diabetes is present, as pointed out in *Expert Opinions in Pharmacotherapy* (November 2001), is to lower blood pressure even more than with high blood pressure alone, namely less than 130/80 mm Hg. If kidney damage has already occurred, the goal pressure is even lower — 125/75 mm Hg to slow down the damage.

The best class of drugs to protect the kidneys and lower blood pressure seems to be the angiotensin-converting enzyme (ACE) inhibitors or the angiotensin II receptor blockers. Their protection goes beyond just lowering blood pressure because other classes of drugs that lower blood pressure to the same extent don't protect the kidneys as well. How they do this isn't clear.

If coronary artery disease is present, then beta-adrenergic blocking agents are the first choice with thiazide diuretics or calcium channel blocking agents as the second choice. Fixed combinations of an ACE inhibitor and a thiazide diuretic or a beta-adrenergic blocking agent may be the best treatment in terms of cost and effectiveness.

Risking High Blood Pressure If You Smoke

An interesting study from Tours, France, in *Journal of Hypertension* (February 2002) shows that people who smoked and then stopped as well as people who currently smoke have a much higher risk of developing high blood pressure than people who never smoked.

Out of 12,417 men, 13.5 percent of those who had quit smoking had high blood pressure. But only 8.8 percent of the men who had never smoked had high blood pressure — regardless of age or tendency to drink alcoholic beverages. Current smokers were also at higher risk for high blood pressure than non-smokers, especially after the age of 60, with a 26 percent risk. The more cigarettes smoked and the greater the duration of smoking, the greater the risk of high blood pressure. The weight of the former smokers, however, seemed to explain the greater prevalence of high blood pressure in this group because the former smokers tended to be heavy. The percentage of high blood pressure among current smokers was independent of their weight.

If you currently smoke, you're likely to have high blood pressure. If you smoked at one time, you're still likely to have high blood pressure. If you don't smoke, then don't ever start!

Another study of smokers and nonsmokers in China in the *Journal of Hypertension* (February 2001) showed that quitting smoking and taking medications had about the same blood pressure-lowering benefit for the patient with high blood pressure. Those who continued to smoke had a much higher risk of a brain attack. Quitting smoking might prevent 51 brain attacks in untreated patients with high blood pressure and 45 additional brain attacks in treated patients with high blood pressure for every 1,000 people with high blood pressure.

Clarifying the Role of Salt

The fact that salt raises blood pressure in salt-sensitive people is well known. However, *how* salt raises the blood pressure isn't completely understood. An article in *Journal of Clinical Hypertension* (January 2002) attempts to explain how this occurs: In the salt-sensitive people, the tissue on the inside of the arteries, called the *endothelium,* is unable to produce the chemical nitric oxide when exposed to excessive salt. Nitric oxide widens blood vessels, which tends to lower blood pressure. Without nitric oxide, the blood pressure rises and, in turn, damages the kidneys, heart, and blood vessels.

Salt may not raise blood pressure in those individuals who don't have salt sensitivity. Controlling salt intake and avoiding increased weight due to salt and water retention makes sense, however, even if you're one of those folks who isn't salt sensitive.

Another study of salt intake in *Revista Clinica Espanola* (November 2001) showed that salt intake was high in patients with high blood pressure who had been previously advised to follow a low-salt diet. This failure to reduce salt intake may explain, in part, the overall poor success rate of controlling high blood pressure. Much of this lack of control of salt intake results from the fact that most of the salt added to our food is not added by us but by food manufacturers.

Reduction of salt intake is an important part of controlling high blood pressure, especially as you get older and become even more salt sensitive. Be aware of all the salt added by food manufacturers by reading food nutrition labels.

Gauging the Impact of Preeclampsia

High blood pressure is one of the symptoms of *preeclampsia,* which is blood poisoning during the latter stages of pregnancy that's thought to result from an inadequate blood flow between the uterus and the placental tissue (see Chapter 16). A Canadian study in the *American Journal of Epidemiology* (February 2002) looked at the consequences for the birth weight of a baby born to women with preeclampsia.

Out of the 97,270 pregnancies, depending on the number of weeks that the fetus was able to remain in the uterus, babies from mothers who had preeclampsia were significantly smaller than those who had normal blood pressure. Mothers with preeclampsia who delivered before 37 weeks had babies who were 352 grams (roughly 12.4 ounces) lighter than mothers who didn't have preeclampsia. If the baby was delivered after 37 weeks, however, the birth weights were the same regardless of the presence of preeclampsia.

The fact that babies who were delivered after 37 weeks of pregnancy were the same weight regardless of whether preeclampsia was present suggests that the cause may not be inadequate blood flow. If preeclampsia was the result of inadequate blood flow, then babies who lasted longer in the uterus with preeclampsia would be expected to be even lighter as compared to those whose mothers didn't have preeclampsia.

Another important aspect of preeclampsia is *cystatin C* — a chemical that was just discovered in the blood per a study in the *Scandinavian Journal of Clinical Laboratory Investigation* (July 2001). Preeclampsia can be associated with kidney damage in the mother. The level of cystatin C in the bloodstream is a better marker for kidney damage in preeclampsia than other compounds, such as creatinine and uric acid, which were used to chart kidney damage in the blood before cystatin C was discovered.

Treating Sleep Apnea

Obstructive sleep apnea (see Chapter 4) is a condition in which a person stops breathing for as long as one minute while sleeping. This one-minute halt may occur five or more times within an hour, and high blood pressure may result when the lack of oxygen causes a constriction of blood vessels. With millions of people suffering from sleep apnea, it may be a major contributor to the prevalence of high blood pressure.

Sleep apnea consists of multiple one-minute breathless periods (ten or more an hour is diagnostic that symptomatic sleep apnea that can raise blood pressure is present). Typically, an individual with sleep apnea may awaken during sleep and gasp for air after breathing has stopped for a minute or less. Although the signs of sleep apnea are clear, probably 80 percent of the people who have it, don't know it. The key questions to ask yourself are

- ✔ Are you excessively sleepy during the day?
- ✔ Does your partner complain about your snoring?
- ✔ Has your partner witnessed that you have episodes of not breathing?

If the answer to these questions is yes, you're a likely candidate for the diagnosis, and your high blood pressure may be related to it. Obstructive sleep apnea is easily diagnosed and treated. If treated early enough, it may help you to avoid irreversible high blood pressure.

An article in the *American Family Physician* (January 2002) discusses the positive consequences of diagnosing and treating sleep apnea. With treatment, the daytime and nighttime blood pressures fall. This may decrease the likelihood of heart complications, not to mention the improved ability to work and drive a car (see Chapter 4). Dramatic improvement in the overall quality of life takes place when patients are successfully treated for obstructive sleep apnea.

According to an article from France in the *New England Journal of Medicine* (February 2002), speeding up the heart while a person sleeps with a device called a *pacemaker* (a device that stimulates the heart to beat at a set rate), the number of episodes of sleep apnea could be reduced from nine to three times an hour. The patients in this study slept just as much as when they did not have their hearts speeded up. The patients with pacemakers felt better, and their blood pressure was lower. This pacemaker technique may be a major new method for preventing high blood pressure in obstructive sleep apnea.

Considering the Role of Ethnic Beliefs

I have repeatedly noted the importance of physical activity to lower blood pressure. An important study in *Preventive Medicine* (February 2002), compares the levels of physical activity among 16,246 adults from various ethnic groups with the prevalence of high blood pressure in those groups.

Among non-Hispanic African Americans, a high rate of high blood pressure exists as compared to other ethnic groups. They had very little leisure time physical activity. The ethnic groups that had the most leisure time physical activity (such as non-Hispanic Caucasians) had the lowest prevalence of high blood pressure after adjusting other factors, such as salt intake, weight, and alcohol intake.

This study emphasizes that to the extent that race is a factor for determining the level of physical activity, race also plays an important role in the occurrence of high blood pressure. Because certain ethnic groups encourage a sedentary life style, those groups tend to have more frequent high blood pressure.

Another study in the *American Journal of Medicine* (January 2002) looked at the ethnic beliefs of African Americans about the origins and treatment of high blood pressure. In Texas, it was discovered that many African Americans believed that high blood pressure was caused by pork or other foods that made the blood travel too fast to the head. These people often believed that vitamins, garlic, and other herbs could treat high blood pressure. Many of them didn't realize that high blood pressure could be a cause of death.

This study concluded that one important reason for the failure of certain groups to control high blood pressure may be the prevalence of beliefs about high blood pressure that are inconsistent with current medical understanding.

Performing Surgery

Because being overweight or obese can bring about high blood pressure, many attempts have been made to help overweight people lose weight and keep it off.

An Australian study in *Diabetes Care* (February 2002) looks at the health consequences of *laparascopic gastric banding,* surgery that makes the stomach smaller with an adjustable band, which limits the amount of food that can be eaten and thus causes weight loss. During the surgery, a small hole is made in the abdomen over the stomach, and a band is attached around the stomach.

A number of positive metabolic and physical results were found in 500 consecutive patients treated in this way. For example, the average weight loss was about 60 pounds. Of the 50 patients with diabetes, 64 percent had a complete loss of high blood glucose levels and 26 percent had major improvements. High blood pressure fell in most of the patients who lost weight. They also showed improvement in their blood fats, including cholesterol and triglycerides. The surgery is not entirely benign since some patients had wound infections or other complications that were successfully managed.

Chapter 20

Ten+ Places to Go for the Latest Information

• •

In This Chapter

▶ Accessing the facts on the Internet

▶ Mailing away for free booklets

• •

A wealth of information about high blood pressure is waiting for you. If you think the riches that the old pirates left on some Caribbean island are vast, just wait until you tap into the riches that many organizations and people provide free of charge to you about high blood pressure. It boggles the mind. Practically all of it's on the Internet. You can read it, download it, print it out, or just stare at it happily. What? You still don't have a connection to the Internet? If you have high blood pressure, the treasure that's on the Internet with respect to this one subject is enough reason to get connected.

If you made up your mind to live and die without ever touching a computer keyboard, another means is available to you for accessing valuable information on the subject of high blood pressure. It's that quaint instrument, the telephone, or failing that, the phenomenon that's now called *snail mail,* which refers to the speed that anything travels when it's carried from place to place. If available, I provide you with an organization's phone number and address in addition to the Web site.

This chapter offers the best of the best — so many great resources for high blood pressure are available that limiting them to just ten is difficult. So at the end of the chapter, I list a few more Web sites that are worth looking at.

How do you know whether a Web site offers authoritative information or unsubstantiated myths? Fortunately, Health On the Net Foundation (HON), an international Swiss organization, has made it their mission to help people like you and me access valid medical and health-related information on the Web. Any Web site with the HON logo has fulfilled the requirements of the HON Code of Conduct:

✔ Only qualified individuals offer medical advice.

✔ The user's identity is kept confidential.

✔ Claims of medical treatment are supported by evidence.

✔ Advertising and editorial information are clearly separated.

HON recognizes all the Web sites in this chapter. If you want to search the HON site for links to the Web addresses that the foundation has evaluated for any medical topic, go to their Web site's index page (www.hon.ch) and enter a keyword to retrieve Web pages. At the next page, you can choose to limit your search to those sites subscribing to the HON Code. For example, using the keyword *hypertension,* I was given a total of 3,081 sites that discussed high blood pressure: 73 sites that subscribed to the code plus 3,008 other sites that didn't.

Starting with the National High Blood Pressure Education Program

The National High Blood Pressure Education Program's Web site (www.nhlbi.nih.gov/hbp) is a great place to start adding to your understanding of high blood pressure. (You can also reach the program at 301-496-4236.) The National Heart, Lung, and Blood Institute started the program in 1972 to create public education programs for the reduction of high blood pressure and its complications.

This site has many resources concerning high blood pressure. On the index page, you can find a selection of 55 topics from ACE inhibitors to hormone replacement therapy to the white coat effect with everything in between. Besides the basic information, tips and quizzes, information about medications and working with your doctor, real-life examples of people with high blood pressure and information about National High Blood Pressure Education Month, which occurs in May each year, are all available. Information on the National High Blood Pressure Education Month can be found on the Internet (http://hin.nhlbi.nih.gov/nhbpep_kit).

If you want information that you can't find at this Web site, follow the links to "Contact NHLBI" where you can get an answer to just about any question on high blood pressure.

Utilizing the U.S National Library of Medicine

The U.S. National Library of Medicine Web site (www.nlm.nih.gov) provides links to MEDLINEplus Health Information and PubMed. (See more on MEDLINEplus and PubMed coming up in this section.) You can also write to the U.S. National Library of Medicine for more information at 8600 Rockville Pike, Bethesda, MD 20894 or call 301-496-6221.

MEDLINEplus Health Information

The MEDLINEplus Health Information Web site (www.medlineplus.gov) contains about 500 discussions of health topics from the National Institutes of Health including high blood pressure. Discussions specific to high blood pressure can be found on the Internet at www.nlm.nih.gov/medlineplus/highbloodpressure.html.

The MEDLINEplus site contains both basic descriptions of high blood pressure and up-to-date information about the latest blood pressure discoveries as well as medical advances in general. When I visited, references to articles about high blood pressure had appeared in medical journals just three days earlier. MEDLINEplus also provides lists of hospitals and physicians by state, a medical encyclopedia and dictionaries, health information in Spanish, extensive information on prescription and nonprescription drugs, health information from newspaper and magazine sources, and links to thousands of clinical trials.

As you would expect from any government site, you won't see any advertisements or endorsements.

If you want to, you can sign up for MEDLINEplus weekly updates, but you have to have an e-mail address.

Don't take my word for it, though. *Consumer Reports,* which is my Bible for reliable consumer information, voted MEDLINEplus the best consumer-health Web site for dependable medical information in their January 2002 issue.

PubMed

The U.S. National Library of Medicine also created the PubMed Web site (www.pubmed.gov). You can search PubMed for whatever term you want. In this case, key in *high blood pressure* and click on *Go.* You'll be presented with thousands of references, many with short descriptions, to medical literature about your subject. If you want to limit your search to certain types of litera- ture, such as reviews of a particular subject within a certain time span, you can click on the word *Limits* and choose the appropriate limits for your search.

The PubMed site is something that can only be used on a computer. That you can access thousands of articles on whatever medical topic you choose with the touch of your finger is amazing. If you want more justification for paying your federal taxes, the government's PubMed site serves that function well.

Getting the Facts from the American Heart and Stroke Associations

The American Stroke Association is a division of the American Heart Association. Both the American Heart Association Web site (`www. americanheart.org`) and the American Stroke Association Web site (`www.strokeassociation.org`) offer extensive information for profes- sionals as well as patients. They provide thousands of pages of information and links to other sites where you can find any resource that exists for high blood pressure and brain attacks (see Chapter 7).

You can also write to the American Heart Association or the American Stroke Association for more information at 7272 Greenville Avenue, Dallas, TX 75231 — they both use the same address. You can call the American Heart Association at 800-242-8721 and the American Stroke Association at 888-478-7653.

The American Heart Association

In 1915, The New York Heart Association began as a group of physicians in New York City who were dedicated to gathering and expanding the available information on heart disease. Other similar groups that had formed through- out the country joined to form the American Heart Association in 1924. It began as a scientific society, but in 1948, the association transformed itself into an agency of professional and nonprofessional volunteers. Its mission is to reduce complications from cardiovascular disease and stroke.

To peruse the association's resources on high blood pressure, go directly to the following URL address: `www.americanheart.org/presenter. jhtml?identifier=2114`. Although some advertising gets in the way of this site, advertisements are clearly differentiated from its excellent medical information, such as a series of questions that you may ask about high blood pressure with extensive answers. You may also find stories of people who've had brain attacks and how they survived. (See Chapter 7 for more on brain attacks.) Statistics are available at this site on every aspect of heart disease.

The American Stroke Association

At the American Stroke Association Web site (www.strokeassociation.org), you can find information about the prevention of brain attacks (see Chapter 7), caring for the person who has a brain attack, medical resources, and just about anything that you need to know to deal with this high blood pressure complication.

The American Stroke Association site also features pen pals, so that a brain attack sufferer can communicate with another person who has had a similar attack. To get there from the main page, click on "Stoke Care" in the left hand column. At the next page, click on "Recovery & Support." At the next page, choose "Stroke Family Support Network." Next, select "Stroke Family Warmline" and choose "Correspond with stroke families" found under Related Items on the right side of this page.

Along with the Web site, the American Stroke Association publishes *Stroke Connection Magazine,* containing articles for people who are recovering from a brain attack. Write to the American Stroke Association (address given earlier in this section) to subscribe to this magazine if you don't have Web access.

Investigating the National Stroke Association

The National Stroke Association Web site (www.stroke.org) describes itself as the one nonprofit organization that's 100 percent devoted to stroke. They provide their "top 8 links" to the most common symptoms, recovery and rehabilitation, stroke risk, what is a stroke, acute treatment, effects of stroke, and stroke survivors and their family. That just about covers what you need to know about brain attacks (see Chapter 7).

You can write to them at National Stroke Association, 9707 East Easter Lane, Englewood, CO 80112 or call them at 800-787-6537.

You can also become a nonprofessional member of the organization and receive *Stroke Smart* magazine. If you're a professional, you can join the

Professional Society and receive the *Journal of Stroke and Cerebrovascular Disease* as well as the journal *Stroke: Clinical Updates.*

One of the most useful features of the National Stroke Association site is the link to Related Web Sites and Products where you can find just about any product that a brain attack victim would need: lifts, walkers, wheelchairs, elevators, ramps, reading and writing aids, products for incontinence and hygiene, special clothing, as well as computers and other communication devices for brain attack victims. From the home page of this Web site, click on

- ✔ **Survivor & Caregiver Resources:** To find valuable information for the loved ones of the brain attack victim, from support groups to life at home: dealing with rehabilitation and how the loved one can help.
- ✔ **Clinical Trials:** Tells you about any ongoing studies of drugs and how you can play a role in the study if you've had a brain attack.

All in all, this site should be the first place to go if you need any information on any aspect of prevention, treatment, and rehabilitation for a brain attack.

Finding a Specialist through the American Society of Hypertension

In 1985, a group of professionals who wanted to organize and promote the advancement of scientific information related to cardiovascular diseases started the American Society of Hypertension, now an organization of over 3,000 medical professionals.

The organization's Web site (www.ash-us.org) offers extensive information about high blood pressure. Although the society doesn't make any recommendations, their Web site provides the names and addresses of specialists in the clinical treatment of high blood pressure who are members of the organization.

You can also write to the American Society of Hypertension at 515 Madison Avenue, Suite 1212, New York, NY 10012, or call the society at 212-644-0650.

You can obtain the society's pamphlet *Understanding Hypertension* from off the Internet or by writing to them. Other important publications from the American Society of Hypertension include the *American Journal of Hypertension* and *Current Concepts in Clinical Hypertension,* a newsletter, both of which are directed towards the professional.

Ordering Literature from the National Institutes of Health

The National Institutes of Health Web site (www.nih.gov) has a pamphlet called *HIGH BLOOD PRESSURE: Treat it for Life,* portions of which can be accessed for free at www.nih.gov/health/hbp-tifl. You'll see four sections: an introduction to high blood pressure, a treatment section, a section on special concerns such as the elderly and diabetics, and resources for more information and a program for exercise.

Among its other useful features are a sample walking program, menu ideas, recipes, and a glossary of terms relating to blood pressure.

The booklet can be purchased in its entirety for five dollars from the U.S. Government Printing Office, Superintendent of Documents, Mail Stop: SSOP, Washington, DC 20402-9328. The number of the publication is ISBN 0-16-045176-0.

Searching through the National Kidney Foundation Web Site

Because the kidneys are among those major organs that may both contribute to high blood pressure and be damaged by it, devoting a site to the kidneys is appropriate. The National Kidney Foundation Web site (www.kidney.org/general) fulfills this need. You can also write to the National Kidney Foundation at 30 East 33rd Street, Suite 1100, New York, NY 10016 or call 1-800-622-9010.

The site contains information about high blood pressure and your kidney. You can search seven categories of information on: health information, donor family support, nutrition, treatment, rehabilitation, and organ donation and healthcare services. If you choose health information, for example, you're presented with about 40 different topics that cover every aspect of disease affecting the kidneys. Many of the topics have to do with both high blood pressure and kidney disease.

The National Kidney Foundation also publishes three different magazines, *Family Focus* for dialysis patients, *Transplant Chronicles* for people who have received a kidney transplant, and *For Those Who Give and Grieve,* a publication for loved ones of organ donors. (Subscribe to these publications by writing to the National Kidney Foundation at the address given earlier in this section.)

Discovering the National Institute of Diabetes & Digestive & Kidney Diseases

The National Institute of Diabetes & Digestive & Kidney Diseases Web site (www.niddk.nih.gov) has valuable information on all aspects of diabetes, gastrointestinal disease, and kidney disease. You can access information specific to high blood pressure and the kidneys at www.niddk.nih.gov/health/kidney/summary/hypotens/hypotens.htm. This area of the site provides information about how high blood pressure damages the kidneys, how you can prevent it, and what to do if kidney damage has already occurred.

This site also has links to numerous publications on all aspects of kidney diseases. For example, a link is available to extensive descriptions of dialysis techniques.

To request information through the mail, write to the U. S. Government Printing Office at Superintendent of Documents, Mail Stop: SSOP, Washington, DC 20402-9328. The organization also offers many of its publications in Spanish.

Consulting with the Mayo Clinic

The world-renowned Mayo Clinic Web site (www.mayoclinic.com) has extensive material on every aspect of disease including high blood pressure. Going to the Mayo Clinic Web site is like having a super easy-to-understand medical textbook. On the Internet at www.mayoclinic.com/findinformation/diseasesandconditions, you can find links to various pages of this same site, other valuable Web sites, and discussions on high blood pressure.

Viewing Lifeclinic.com

Lifeclinic.com has extensive information about three major health disorders: high blood pressure, high cholesterol, and diabetes. Simply key in the Lifeclinic Web site (www.lifeclinic.com) and explore.

Although you see some advertising, this site follows the HON Code of Conduct. It goes through basic facts about high blood pressure and then how to lower it. The site tells you how to monitor your blood pressure and the risk factors for heart disease. You can also locate discussions on low blood pressure, high blood pressure and pregnancy, brain attacks (see Chapter 7), and heart failure at this site.

One of the nice features of the site is the ability to keep a health record that can be accessed from any computer with the proper identification and password. You can keep records of your blood pressure, pulse, weight, cholesterol, blood sugar, personal health records, family health records, and a health checklist.

If you have a health question, you can ask the experts. An extensive directory of medicines is also available where you can find everything that you need to know about a medication including what it does, adverse reactions, drug interactions, how to take it, and how to store it.

A physician directory is also available on this Web site so that patients with high blood pressure can find a physician online. Furthermore, it offers Web site reviews, book reviews, patient pamphlets, topics regarding high blood pressure, and the latest news. You can also find a cookbook filled with healthy recipes with a list of all the sources of kilocalories and the amount of nutrients for that recipe.

Lifeclinic.com has set up 11,700 Health Stations in retail stores where you can get health information. Lifeclinic.com has won numerous awards for the quality of its material. You'll benefit both from the information on this site and the many services offered.

Checking Other Sites

Some other useful Web sites include the following:

- Focus on High Blood Pressure at `www.focusonhighbloodpressure.com`.
- Visit Dr. Blood Pressure at `www.drbloodpressure.com`.
- See WebMD Health at `www.health.medscape.com/highbloodpressurecenter`.
- Go to Blood Pressure.Com at `www.bloodpressure.com`.
- Discover the DASH diet at the National Institutes of Health Web page `www.nhlbi.nih.gov/health/public/heart/hbp/dash`.

If you live outside the United States, some of the best sources of information about high blood pressure can be found at the following addresses:

- ✔ United Kingdom: Patient UK at `www.patient.co.uk/illness/b/blood_pressure.htm`

- ✔ Australia: The National Heart Foundation of Australia at `www.heartfoundation.com.au`

- ✔ Canada: The Canadian Coalition for High Blood Pressure Prevention and Control at `www.canadianbpcoalition.org/english/links.htm`

- ✔ Other countries: The World Hypertension League at `www.mco.edu/org/whl/northam.html#us`

Index

ERT (estrogen replacement therapy),
260–262, 289
erythropoietin, 87, 279
ESRD. *See* end-stage renal disease
essential high blood pressure
  elderly, 229
  explanation of, 12, 36
  kidney, 88–89
estrogen replacement therapy (ERT),
260–262, 289
ethacrynic acid, 195
ethnicity, 32–34
etodolac, 231
exercise
  aerobic exercise, 174–176
  anaerobic exercise, 174
  benefits, 172
  biking, 176
  children, 248–249
  clothing, 176
  cross-training, 274
  equipment, 176, 274
  frequency, importance of, 176–177
  heart attack, 81
  high cholesterol, 79
  lowering blood pressure with, 12,
    39–40, 122, 171–176, 273–274
  myths about, 286–287
  New Year's Resolution exerciser, 273
  Perceived Exertion Scale, 177
  physical condition, checking, 173
  during pregnancy, 254
  role of race in determining levels of, 298
  strength training, 178–180
  walking, 174–175
  weight lifting, 178–180, 274
  weight loss, 177–178
  Yoga, 181
exercise electrocardiogram, 173
Expert Opinions in Pharmacotherapy, 294
exudate, 89

eyes
  blindness, 89
  blurred vision, symptom of stroke, 106
  cotton wool spots, 105
  diabetic retinopathy, 46
  exudate, 89
  funduscopic examination, 105
  malignant high blood pressure, 89
  papilledema, 89
  white spots, 89

• F •

Family Caregiver Alliance, 113
Family Focus magazine, 307
family history, role in high blood
    pressure, 31–32
fasting, 138
FDA (Food and Drug Administration),
    186
Feldene, 231
felodipine, 210
Feuerstein, Georg (*Yoga For Dummies*),
    181
fibromuscular disease, 48
finding a doctor, 306, 309
Fitness For Dummies (Liz Neporent and
    Suzanne Schlosberg), 172
fixed-dose combinations of medications,
    293–294
Focus on High Blood Pressure Web site,
    309
Food and Drug Administration (FDA),
    186
food label
  low-salt food, 146
  nutrition facts, 147, 272
food
  additives, 145
  cardiovascular system, 10
  DASH diet, 130–132
  high-salt food, 147